MANAGING SUICIDAL RISK

Managing Suicidal Risk

A Collaborative Approach

DAVID A. JOBES

Foreword by Edwin S. Shneidman

THE GUILFORD PRESS
New York   London

Printed in the United States of America

This book is printed on acid-free paper.

Last digit is print number: 9 8 7 6 5 4 3 2

Library of Congress Cataloging-in-Publication Data

Jobes, David A.
    Managing suicidal risk : a collaborative approach / by David A. Jobes.
       p. cm.
    Includes bibliographical references and index.
    ISBN-10: 1-59385-327-0   ISBN-13: 978-1-59385-327-3 (pbk.)
    1. Suicide.   I. Title.
    RC569.J63 2006
    362.28—dc22

                                                                          2006004985

To Colleen, Connor, and Dillon
and to the memory of
Frank S. Jobes and Steven D. Jobes

About the Author

David A. Jobes, PhD, is a Professor of Psychology at The Catholic University of America, where he is also the Codirector of Clinical Training of the PhD clinical psychology program. With research interests in suicidology, he has published extensively in the field and routinely conducts professional training in clinical suicidology. Dr. Jobes is a consultant to the U.S. Air Force Suicide Prevention Program and is a clinical consultant to the Psychology Service of the Washington, DC, Veterans Affairs Medical Center. He has served as a consultant to various Washington, DC, area counseling centers, the Centers for Disease Control and Prevention, and the Institute of Medicine of the National Academy of Sciences. Dr. Jobes is Associate Editor for the journal *Suicide and Life-Threatening Behavior*. He is a past president, treasurer, and board member of the American Association of Suicidology (AAS) and is a recipient of the AAS Edwin S. Shneidman Award in recognition of early career contributions to suicidology. As a board-certified clinical psychologist (American Board of Professional Psychology), Dr. Jobes maintains a private clinical and forensic practice at the Washington Psychological Center.

Foreword

It seems as though I have been waiting for a legitimate opportunity to praise David Jobes in print, for I have admired his work, his thinking, and his professional style for many years. For some time I have considered him one of my favorite suicidologists of "the second generation." (He is in the age range of my own four sons, who are also health professionals.) David's book about the Collaborative Assessment and Management of Suicidality (CAMS) is like Mozart to my ears, especially so in the way that it captures and extends some of my own ideas about the nature of the suicidal mind.

This useful book is a roadmap through the land of pain and suffering—psychache—that is unique to the suicidal person. Many people suffer; many people are in pain. But suicide belongs to psychache. No psychache, no suicide. I am most pleased that *psychache* and my related constructs of psychological *press* and *perturbation* are the central conceptual foundation of the CAMS approach. I am further delighted to note that the Suicide Status Form (SSF)—the core assessment tool used in CAMS—is built around the Cubic Model of Suicide that was presented over 20 years ago in *The Definition of Suicide* (Shneidman, 1985). Obviously, Jobes has a particularly keen eye for good ideas.

As a clinician-researcher, David Jobes well understands the central importance of listening to the words of suicidal patients as they paint and embellish the picture of psychological suffering that is unique to the suicidal mind. The case examples that are described throughout this book reflect a thoughtfulness about the struggle and a degree of clinical insight that is rare.

David Jobes shares my philosophical love of phenomenology and mentalism. As an academic suicidologist, he has been a tireless researcher with important and scholarly publications. He is a dedicated teacher of students and professionals alike. I take pride in noting that he is a past president of the American Association of Suicidology (AAS) and Associate Editor of the AAS journal, *Suicide and Life-Threatening Behavior*—both close to my heart.

The author shares my deep respect for psychological assessment and testing. His SSF is special among suicide assessment tools as it integrates both quantitative and qualitative methods of clinical assessment. For example, the SSF uses various incomplete sentence blanks prompting suicidal patients to describe in their own written words the exact content and nature of their psychological pain, press, perturbation, hopelessness, and self-hate. It is an imaginative adaptation of the projective technique first developed by Julian Rotter, which speaks volumes about what exactly is on the mind of the suicidal patient. Of course, there are biological and societal considerations in the words of these patients. But what the data show is that more central to their descriptions of suicidal suffering are psychological issues—suicidal mentations related to work and love.

The clinical implications of this book are quite significant. CAMS is a particular approach for understanding and engaging a suicidal mind; it brings an important philosophical orientation to the table of this work. Specifically, CAMS eschews a Kraepelinian approach to understanding a suicidal person as merely a diagnostic specimen in the petri dish of the DSM. Instead, CAMS favors the importance of taking the perspective of the other. The earnest clinical endeavor to empathically understand the suicidal patient's suffering leads to a special therapeutic moment between the patient and therapist—a clinical alliance that enables the pair to get on with addressing the psychache that imperils the patient's life.

My objectivity about this work may be biased and perhaps I exaggerate the scope and importance of this accomplishment. But as an old suicidologist, I recognize when someone comes along and gets it right, speaking essential truths about a topic that I have dedicated my life to understanding.

There is essential clinical wisdom here, informed by empirical data, experience, theory, and pragmatism. Simply stated, this book is an important tool for any clinician who aspires to engage the suicidal mind and clinically venture forth into the world of psychache. This book is good news for the clinician and even better news for the lives of patients this approach will save.

EDWIN S. SHNEIDMAN, PhD
Professor Emeritus of Thanatology
University of California, Los Angeles

Preface

My professional identify is that of a *clinician-researcher*. My entire career since graduate school has been defined by an intentional effort to straddle the perspectives of clinicians in the trenches (seeing real cases in real settings) with the perspectives of researchers (who find their truths in data and laboratories). With our field so divided between these worldviews, I have worked in a determined manner through my career to integrate the truths of *both* perspectives. The critical need for a sound means of clinically assessing and working with the suicidal patient has been all too evident to me from the time I started as a new psychologist and supervisor at the Catholic University Counseling Center in 1987. Consequently, I enthusiastically delved into the research literature to find the best information on clinical work with suicidal patients. Because I had developed an assessment tool in my dissertation (Jobes, Casey, Berman, & Wright, 1991), I was particularly preoccupied with finding a good clinical suicide assessment tool that we could import into our center for regular use with suicidal patients. But as I learned more about the literature in clinical suicidology, I was amazed by how anecdotal, case driven, and nonempirical the literature in this area was (Jobes, 1995a). In other words, the literature of 1980s left me short. Nothing I was reading about working with suicidal patients was really sufficient in addressing the significant demands and particular needs of our patients or our clinical setting.

As I searched for answers to the suicidal clinical challenges we faced in our center, I fortuitously became involved in a survey study that was partially funded by a small grant from the American Association of Suicidology (AAS). This research ultimately culminated in a paper with important findings about how clinicians actually assess suicide risk in real-world settings (Jobes, Eyman, & Yufit, 1995; see also work by Engleman, Jobes, Berman, & Langbein, 1998).

In summary, our survey study found that (1) clinicians in our sample used suicide-specific risk assessment tools relatively rarely; (2) ratings of the utility of suicidal risk assessment measures were relatively low; and (3) among psychologists only (the discipline that is specifically trained in testing), psychological testing overall was relatively more commonly used, but psychological testing was not rated as useful for assessing suicidal risk per se. However, we did find that clinicians liked interview-based questions and liked making behavioral observations to assess suicidal risk.

While these findings may seem obvious, we were actually quite surprised by some of the results. For example, one survey question queried about issues that clinicians might have about using suicide risk assessment tools. A majority of the sample asserted that the limited psychometric properties (i.e., the reliability and validity) of these tools were too problematic. This opinion is curious when one considers the preferred assessment approach of the sample—*clinical interviewing*—as if there is any empirical support for the reliability and validity of this approach to assessment in general clinical practice! Clearly the survey was giving us some insight about human nature.

My overall impression from the risk assessment survey was that clinicians do in fact want to find effective ways for assessing suicide risk. But the data from the survey plainly showed that the available suicide risk assessment tools listed on our questionnaire were neither being used nor clinically valued. I was puzzled. Why were clinicians apparently not interested in using these tools that I thought were so interesting and potentially useful? After a lot of discussions with clinicians in practice, I concluded that there were at least four feasible explanations: (1) a pervasive reliance on—and overconfidence in—clinical interviewing; (2) widespread clinician perceptions that suicide risk assessment tools are impractical (i.e., such tools are seen as clinically intrusive or simply too long); (3) most of the existing instruments are atheoretical; clinicians often do not know the treatment implications or meaning of an obtained risk score; and (4) the common perception that these instruments fail to fundamentally capture essential but elusive aspects of suicidality (Jobes et al., 2004).

In reflecting on the existing roster of available tools both then and now, one can only be struck that almost all of them have been constructed through a multivariate "reductionistic" methodology, what I have elsewhere described as a "top-down" approach to test construction (Jobes et al., 2004). This approach essentially involves taking a large number of psychosocial correlates of completed suicide, suicide attempts, or suicidal ideation, and through multivariate data analyses reducing them to smaller subsets of items that then can be used to constitute the derived assessment scales. It occurred to me that perhaps the key to constructing a new and better tool would be found in taking an entirely different approach to the problem.

With this insight, I set about developing the Suicide Status Form (SSF) over a 15-year period. Ultimately, clinical use and research led to the administration of the SSF within a particular process of clinical engagement and care, which became the Collaborative Assessment and Management of Suicidality—"CAMS" for short. A more detailed discussion of developing and describing the SSF and its use within the CAMS approach is considered in Chapter 2. However, before we more fully consider the clinical research that led to the development of the SSF and CAMS, it is important to have a larger context for this line of work. By understanding the relevant history and background of contemporary clinical suicidology, one can better appreciate why there was a need to develop the CAMS approach as it relates to the current clinical care of suicidal patients.

Finally, it is worth noting that the main title of this book—*Managing Suicidal Risk*—has a double meaning. It is my premise that clinical work with suicidal patients is best performed by collaboratively managing the issue *with the patient*; in turn, such an approach makes the whole challenge of working with suicidal risk much more manageable *for the clinician*. CAMS can be quickly learned and readily used with new cases, or with ongoing cases, whenever suicidal risk is present. It is not meant to be a standalone treatment, but rather serves as a practical method that can be added to one's standard treatment approach—a sensible new tool to be added to any mental health professional's existing therapeutic tool belt.

Acknowledgments

This book on the Collaborative Assessment and Management of Suicidality (CAMS) is the culmination of 20 years of clinical work and research with suicidal patients. Although it is not a final word on this topic, this book is an important milestone in an ongoing line of clinically informed empirical research. There have been many contributors to this line of work worthy of acknowledgment.

While CAMS was born and shaped out of my own clinical experience (which in turn guided the research), the work in this book was largely a direct by-product of Suicide Status Form (SSF) and CAMS research performed with dozens of Catholic University graduate and undergraduate students. The key student contributors (listed chronologically) include Carolyn Eddins, Stephanie Judd, Paula DiCanio, Jennifer Crumlish, Lisa Hustead, Rose Rice, Shawn Bergman, Vanessa Downing, Kristen Francini, Katherine Nelson, Dan Pentiuc, Erin Peterson, Amy Conrad, Steve Wong, Tim Fratto, Vanessa Tendick, Ellen Kahn-Greene, Kyle Grohmann, Mira Brancu, Melinda Moore, and Stephen O'Connor. I would particularly like to acknowledge former students Aaron Jacoby, Jason Luoma, and Rachel Mann, who were the key contributors at the very start of developing CAMS. They were my coauthors on the first iteration of many CAMS manuals that preceded the writing of this book.

There have been many other professional colleagues who have made important contributions and provided critical support, including John Drozd, Diane Arnkoff, George Bonanno, Mark Oordt, Barry Wagner, Marc Sebrechts, Rick Campise, Tracy Neal-Walden, Greg Brown, Michael Mond, Marc Weinstein, Larry David, Peter Cimbolic, John Parkhurst, Diane DePalma, Steve Stein, Israel

Orbach, Konrad Michel, Michael Bostwick, Tim Lineberry, Antoon Leenaars, Rory O'Connor, Keith Hawton, Mark Williams, Thomas Joiner, Kate Comtois, and Morton Silverman. A special thanks goes out to the generous and guiding influences of Lanny Berman, Terry Maltsberger, Marsha Linehan, Aaron Beck, and Ed Shneidman. My colleague David Rudd deserves special acknowledgment for his contributions to the ideas in this book and his unwavering support of me and CAMS.

I am grateful to The Guilford Press; I have appreciated Editor-in-Chief Seymour Weingarten's enthusiastic interest in this project. My Senior Editor at Guilford, Jim Nageotte, has used a remarkably steady hand in shaping this book (and dealing with me). His intelligence, experience, and ideas about developing this book have been incredibly valuable to me.

Throughout my life the support and love of my family—Steve and Bill and my parents, Frank and Helen—has been a constant. My multitalented wife, Colleen, has gone over every word of this book and served as my key "in-house" copy editor, demonstrating editorial skill, intelligence, good humor, unparalleled common sense, and patience with the author. She has taught me a great deal about the true nature of collaboration. When I reflect on my many blessings and what makes my own life so worth living, the list begins with Colleen—our boys, Connor and Dillon—and the family life we have created together.

Finally, I must acknowledge the suicidal patients I have seen over the last 20 years. It is an understatement to say that I have been humbled by their life-and-death struggles. Without question, these patients have taught me the most important lessons I have to impart in this book. These suffering souls have shown me what it takes to struggle and persevere in the face of seemingly unbearable psychological pain. These patients have shown me the formidable seduction of suicide as a kind of psychological undertow that often seems impossible to resist. However, most importantly, these patients have also revealed to me the kind of courage, conviction, and fortitude that it ultimately takes to be able to fight for their lives.

Contents

Contents

CHAPTER 1

Contemporary Clinical Challenges and the Need for Collaborative Assessment and Management of Suicidality

We are in the midst of very challenging times in our efforts to provide competent contemporary mental health care. This is particularly true as it relates to working with suicidal patients. When I first began graduate school in 1982, I took a job as a mental health worker on a nursing staff. The setting was an adult locked inpatient unit in a private psychiatric hospital in a Washington, D.C., suburb located in Maryland. On the second day of my new job, a newly admitted patient made a very severe suicide attempt. Having signed out a pair of scissors from the "sharps" closet, ostensibly to trim his beard, the patient proceeded to stab himself in the throat and abdomen with these very scissors. The nursing staff responded quickly to the dull thud of his body hitting the floor in his bathroom, which was fortuitously located on the other side of the wall from where we were hearing the morning nursing report. The delirious patient who was gushing blood was immediately rushed to a nearby emergency room and was miraculously saved thanks to the quick response of my nursing staff colleagues and the skill of the surgical team. For me it was a horrifying and instructive experience—welcome to the field.

As an aspiring future clinical psychologist, I was filled with idealism and a desire to help others. At the relatively tender professional age of 23, I had extraordinarily naive notions about life-threatening psychological pain and suffering of

1

this magnitude. That morning I found that I was truly appalled that anyone—including a psychotically depressed psychiatric inpatient—could perform such a horrific assault upon his or her own body. It was simply beyond my comprehension. But with no real sense of how, I was nevertheless determined to help this severely depressed man find a way to live.

Keep in mind in 1982 the circumstances of helping such a patient were quite different than the circumstances of today. Within our inpatient psychiatric unit all patients received both intensive group psychotherapy *and* individual psychotherapy along with activity therapies (e.g., art therapy and psychodrama). Patients routinely received full psychological test batteries. Every patient entering into our therapeutic milieu worked his or her way up through four levels of therapeutic care—with associated privileges and freedoms—that were monitored by staff and routinely discussed every morning in unit-wide community meetings. In sharp contrast to contemporary care, malpractice litigation was quite rare, not routine, the range of medicines were still largely first-generation antidepressants (there were no selective serotonin reuptake inhibitors [SSRIs]), and no one yet resented managed care, which would not ascend to dominate health care delivery for some years to come. All these considerations should provide a bit of context for understanding this seminal case experience.

After the patient was medically stabilized, he was promptly transferred back to our unit and given every restriction imaginable (e.g., no use of "sharps," 24-hour-a-day arm's-length constant observation, no street cloths, no visitors, complete restriction to the unit—everything we could do to ensure his safety). Within our first-rate psychiatric facility we helped this patient recover the life he came so close to taking—a treatment that lasted *10 months!* With the steady help of his doctor and our staff we all worked very hard to help him. He dutifully took his medications, attended therapy sessions, and met regularly with his primary nursing staff member and the social worker. This patient endured incredibly difficult moments. I recall one night shift when we chatted at 3:00 A.M. in the bathroom as I sat within arm's length ("constant observation") while he ignominiously had a bowel movement. He met his doctor every morning for psychotherapy at 8:10 A.M. sharp. Various medicines were tried and discarded before the right cocktail of drugs emerged. He met with his wife and children in family therapy conducted by a skilled family therapist.

Eventually, with a quiet sense of dignified determination and the magic mix of the right combination of medications and therapies, this severely depressed man worked his way off all the various and severe restrictions that were placed on him. With a growing sense of resolve and even the traces of a budding confidence that imperceptibly evolved over days, weeks, and months, this patient climbed the ladder of our levels system, rung by rung, finding both a therapeutic stride and a sense of real recovery within our therapeutic milieu. This painstaking process of growth and progress was associated with increased privileges. Eventually there were a series of passes that began with short hourly passes and progressed to overnight passes. Much to our mutual joy he was subsequently discharged from our unit, returning to home and family. Both literally and figuratively scarred forever by his brutal suicidal act, he nevertheless survived the horrors of that morning, to return to the joys—and challenges—of home, family, and work.

While perhaps a relatively dramatic case example, the treatment aspects of this influential professional experience were consistent with standard psychiatric care of the early 1980s. Indeed, unlike today, it was not at all uncommon in that era for a depressed and suicidal patient to be hospitalized for weeks, months, even *years.* Moreover, patients with even mild or passing suicidal thoughts were routinely hospitalized; in fact, even patients with *no* suicidal thoughts at all could still be hospitalized for lengthy stays.

Clearly, times have changed since my experience in 1982. As psychiatric inpatient hospitalization lengths of stay have plummeted since the early 1990s, it is not uncommon for an inpatient hospitalization stay to be as short as 3 to 4 days (Olfson, Gameroff, Marcus, Greenberg, & Shaffer, 2005); other data suggest an average that ranges from 6 to 10 days (Figueroa, Harman, & Engberg, 2004; National Alliance for the Mentally Ill, 2000). My own sense is that mean lengths of stay may be somewhat misleading, whereas I suspect modes of hospital stays may be a truer index of remarkably short psychiatric hospital stays. Whatever the case, undoubtedly lengths of stay are markedly different from 1990 when the average psychiatric hospitalization was 25.6 days (National Alliance for the Mentally Ill, 2000). These days most psychiatric hospitalizations are *necessarily* related to acute suicidal risk. In my own experience, admissions for patients without suicidal risk have become quite rare. Once admitted the suicidal inpatient must remain highly suicidal to stay in the hospital. But in this regard, many mental health professionals perceive that pressures to quickly discharge psychiatric inpatients are all too often driven by purely economic considerations rather than by a true clinical abatement of the suicidal risk.

This sequence of steps in contemporary inpatient care now ultimately leads us to the peculiar—and in my view problematic—use of "safety contracts" or "no-suicide contracts" wherein nursing staff typically compel patients to promise (even having them sign a written form) that they will not hurt themselves until their next designated outpatient appointment. As discussed further in Chapter 5, the problem with contemporary use of safety contracts is that they are neither about safety nor truly contractual in any legal sense. Yet, they are pervasively used all over the country and probably reflect routine care. In truth, however, safety contracts are all too often used very inappropriately—as a mere ploy or maneuver to move the patient along while still providing the appearance of "protective" documentation within the clinical record. Nevertheless, in my experience as a forensic expert, safety contracts often come back to haunt clinician-defendants rather than "protecting" them from malpractice litigation because the contract obviously failed to protect the patient from a suicidal demise.

Based on case descriptions and questions I receive from clinicians in general practice, I have concluded the following: A suicidal patient equals threat and trouble; therefore, inpatient hospitalization equals safety and decreased trouble (i.e., no liability). But these perceptions begin to shift and change when a clinician actually engages an insurance carrier in an attempt to precertify a suicidal patient for inpatient care (a unique battle unto itself). Indeed, one clinician in Des Moines told me that he tried to hospitalize a highly suicidal patient only to learn that acute suicidal *ideation* was not sufficient to precertify an inpatient hospitalization if it is not accompanied by an attempt *behavior* (i.e., imminent ideation may not be enough to hospitalize). Whatever the case, if the erstwhile and determined clinician "wins" the precertification battle with the insurance company and actually succeeds in getting a patient into the hospital, the clinician is often shocked to find the attending psychiatrist or the clinical social worker calling the *next* day to discuss discharge and outpatient disposition. In addition, the patient is often angry and hostile about the hospitalization experience, feeling like a few days in the hospital has not improved the situation but actually made matters worse. I have a patient that I still see who I hospitalized over 10 years ago. She still counts her 4-day inpatient experience as one of the most devastating events of her life (even though she readily acknowledges that it may well have saved her from a seriously suicidal state).

Many of the various changes in contemporary psychiatry and mental health care can be directly attributed to the explosion of research and development of new psychotropic medications. One of the obvious virtues of pharmacological treatments is that it they are remarkably cheap—a compelling consideration in an era of managed health care. The downside to medication-based treatment of course is that patients must actually behaviorally *take* their medications as prescribed and attend follow-up appointments with their doctors for these drugs to optimally work. But as I have discussed elsewhere (Jobes & Drozd, 2004), typical outpatient compliance behaviors related to taking medication is often abysmal, and a patients' apparent ability to attend follow-up appointments is often woefully inadequate.

Add to these considerations the very real prospect of poor treatment outcomes and the situation gets even more complex. Obviously poor outcomes in the case of suicidality may include potentially significant injury due to a failed attempt, or in a worst-case scenario, death. It follows within our incredibly litigious society that when things go badly with suicide related behaviors, legal action often quickly follows. Indeed, recent research has shown that it has become virtually axiomatic that surviving family members will either consider contacting an attorney to pursue malpractice litigation after a loved one in treatment dies by suicide (Luoma, Martin, & Pearson, 2002). A few decades ago, only inpatient facilities (and providers) were sued for malpractice. But as I noted over 10 years ago, the risk of malpractice litigation against *outpatient* mental health providers has increased exponentially and this litigation costs malpractice insurance carriers a great deal of money (Jobes & Berman, 1993).

From my vantage point as a career suicidologist, the extraordinary confluence of societal, economic, professional, psychotherapeutic, pharmacological, and legal changes over the past two decades has left many contemporary clinicians without a safety net for their patients or themselves—they frankly do not know what to do with these cases and many of them are scared. The relative comfort that clinicians had enjoyed some years ago—that they could safely hospitalize a patient for as long as was needed—has essentially disappeared, most likely *forever*. I have encountered countless clinicians who say with great apprehension and shame that they have lost a patient to suicide and now face the horrors of malpractice litigation. I have seen still other clinicians with fear in their eyes, not knowing how to proceed with a life-and-death suicidal case that is making them feel desperate and incompetent. I have battled with insurance personnel to precertify patients for hospitalization only to have those very patients discharged the next morning by the attending doctor over my vigorous objections. In one case an attending doctor actually told my patient, "The next time you feel like overdosing on your medication, just don't do it." She readily promised to do so and he discharged her back to my outpatient care. In the next 3 years she repeatedly broke her promise and proceeded to overdose another three times.

These anecdotes and experiences are not unique; many clinicians have gone through similar and related experiences. Like me they have felt helpless and sometimes even incompetent when working with seriously suicidal patients. They know that contemporary hospitalization can be quite limited; medications can only do so much, and if they lose a patient to suicide it is likely that malpractice litigation against them will at least be considered if not actively pursued. We clinicians today face considerable issues and challenges when we encounter a suicidal patient. Clearly there is a need for a novel approach that is fundamentally designed to address them. This book is dedicated to presenting such a method. The Collaborative Assessment and Management of Suicidality (CAMS) is both a specific clinical approach and a philosophy for working with suicidal patients that was derived, shaped, and formed out of pragmatic clinical need.

WHAT IS CAMS AND HOW DOES IT WORK?

CAMS is an overall process of clinical assessment, treatment planning, and management of suicidal risk with suicidal outpatients. The CAMS process of care has three distinct phases: (1) initial "Index" Assessment/Treatment Planning, (2) Clinical Tracking, and (3) Clinical Outcomes. In other words, the process of CAMS has a beginning, a middle, and an end. The core multipurpose tool used within all the CAMS phases is the SSF. The seven pages of the SSF serve as a *roadmap* for guiding the clinician and patient through CAMS, providing crucial documentation along the way pertaining to each of the three phases of clinical care with a suicidal patient. The specific clinical procedures of CAMS are discussed in great detail in Chapters 3–7. However, beyond the specific clinical procedures of CAMS there are important philosophical issues in relation to our discussion of contemporary clinical care of the suicidal patient that are useful to consider as we bring this particular chapter to a close.

CAMS AS A CLINICAL PHILOSOPHY

Philosophically, CAMS as a clinical approach is fundamentally oriented toward keeping suicidal patients *out* of inpatient hospital settings. CAMS patients are quickly and directly engaged in the clinical assessment of their suicidal risk. Moreover, suicidal patients are further engaged through CAMS in the management of their own outpatient safety and stability. CAMS provides structure—it is a therapeutic framework—that guides *both* parties through the assessment and subsequent clinical care. CAMS is a process—it creates a therapeutic vehicle that enables the clinician and patient to travel over some rocky (suicidal) roads together. Use of the SSF within CAMS enables both parties to examine the patient's suicidality in a relatively objective manner—how suicide has become compelling to the patient as a means of coping. But in this shared understanding there is always the potential that suicidal coping can be replaced with alternative ways of coping. Within the CAMS approach, the formation of a strong and viable clinical alliance is central. Moreover, CAMS is designed to fundamentally optimize the *patient's* motivation. Treatment theory and empirical research has clearly shown that these variables (clinical alliance + high patient motivation) are essential to good clinical outcomes (Garfield, 1994; Horvath & Symonds, 1991; Overholser, 2005). By maximizing the alliance and patient motivation, CAMS helps the patient find alternative ways of coping with the help of mental health care. Within CAMS, suicidal patients learn to rely on their clinician; in turn they learn to rely on *themselves* as they find better ways to cope and problem-solve. When coping and problem solving improves, the option of suicide can be made systematically obsolete through thoughtful and systematic clinical care that is central to the CAMS approach.

We intuitively know that human beings have struggled and emotionally suffered since the beginning of time. Indeed, some people suffer so much that the concept of taking their life seems to be the only option to end the pain. For my part, I am interested in giving these people an opportunity to make their seemingly unlivable lives, somehow livable. Bottom line, what we know to be most true about the vast majority of people who kill themselves can be boiled down to three essential truisms:

- Most suicidal people do not want an end to their biological existence; rather, they want an end to their psychological pain and suffering.
- Most suicidal people tell others (including mental professionals) that they are thinking about suicide as a compelling option for coping with their pain.
- Most suicidal people have psychological problems, social problems, and poor methods for coping with pain—all things that mental health professionals are usually well trained to tackle.

Clearly, suicidal people are searching for an option and they often need help if they are to find an alternative to suicide. In turn, we clinicians through our professional training and experiences are uniquely positioned to create alternative options and provide life-saving help to our patients. To that end, I am passionately interested in providing a reasonable response to ending psychological pain without costing a patient his or her life. I have heard what my suicidal patients have said about their pain and suffering and I am dedicated to responding effectively to that pain and suffering. I am especially resolved to use my training and skills to fundamentally address psychological and social problems, creating whole new and better ways of coping with seemingly unbearable pain. Responding to these three truisms is what CAMS is all about. Helping our patients to find a way to choose life is the point of all our efforts in this most crucial of all clinical endeavors.

CHAPTER 2

A Review of the Suicide Status Form and the Origin of CAMS

Now that we have a bit of context for understanding the need for CAMS, let us pick up our discussion from the Preface about the initial pragmatic clinical need to develop a novel assessment tool that clinicians would actually use. This practical notion—developing reasonable and usable clinical approaches to suicidality—has been a guiding idea since the inception of my empirical work on the Suicide Status Form (SSF). Similarly, practical considerations and clinical utility further shaped the empirical work that ultimately led to the development of the larger CAMS approach right to the present day. This line of clinically driven research originally began in 1988 with the initial development of the SSF. Because the SSF is so central to the use of CAMS, this chapter initially provides a detailed discussion of the development of the SSF and a thorough review of each component part of the form. The chapter then concludes with the ultimate application of the SSF as it is used within the CAMS approach. As I show, it was the particular application of the SSF tool within the larger CAMS framework and philosophy that marked the genesis of this novel clinical approach to suicidality.

THE SSF

The SSF was purposely designed to achieve a variety of different goals (beyond assessment), which sets it apart from many of the existing suicide risk assessment tools. As will become clear, the SSF was constructed to be versatile and have multiple applications as it is used within the larger CAMS approach. Just to be extra clear on this point: The SSF is the core multipurpose tool that is used within the larger clinical assessment and management process called the Collaborative Assessment and Management of Suicidality. Thus, within the CAMS approach, the SSF is used to:

1. Conduct and document a multidimensional collaborative assessment of the suicidal patient's initial suicidal risk.
2. Collaboratively develop and document a suicide-specific treatment plan for the suicidal patient.
3. Clinically track and document ongoing suicidal risk as well as note any updates to the suicidal patient's treatment plan.
4. Determine and document clinical outcomes when CAMS is concluded.

Because the SSF is so central to using the CAMS approach it is important to thoroughly review each component part in depth to appreciate the multipurpose nature of the form. As noted earlier and shown in Appendix A, the full SSF is made up of seven different pages that are divided into three phases of clinical care: (1) Index Assessment/Treatment Planning (SSF pages 1–3), (2) Clinical Tracking (SSF pages 4–5), and (3) Clinical Outcomes (SSF pages 6–7). Thus, there are three distinct phases of SSF used within the process of using CAMS with any suicidal patient (i.e., there are distinct phases that include a beginning, a middle, and an end).

In the beginning, the Index Assessment/Treatment Planning session is conducted with any *currently* identified suicidal patient (i.e., anyone who is immediately suicidal or has been so in the past seven days). This first phase of CAMS requires the use of the first three SSF pages, which are divided into four distinct sections (Sections A–D). After the index session there are typically a series of clinical tracking sessions for a suicidal patient who is referred to being on "Suicide Status," which is an administrative descriptor of CAMS patients who have ongoing suicidal risk. The second phase of CAMS—Clinical Tracking—requires the use of SSF pages 4 and 5; these tracking pages are divided into three distinct sections (Sections A–C). As discussed in further depth in Chapter 6, suicidal patients within CAMS may be on Suicide Status for as short as three postindex tracking sessions or for many tracking sessions if they do not reach criteria for resolution or other clinical outcomes. For all Suicide Status tracking sessions, SSF pages 4 and 5 are repeatedly used. The third phase of CAMS—Clinical Outcomes— requires the use of SSF pages 6 and 7, which are divided into three distinct sections (Sections A–C). These forms are used to bring CAMS to conclusion when certain criteria are met or other outcomes are realized.

In summary, the SSF is the core assessment, treatment planning, tracking, and outcome clinical tool used within the CAMS. The seven pages of the SSF are used as a *roadmap* for guiding the three phases of CAMS—Index Assessment/Treatment Planning, Clinical Tracking, and Clinical Outcomes. Given the multipurpose use of the SSF, the following discussion traverses the entire seven-page SSF document further clarifying the three phases of CAMS while simultaneously discussing the clinical process and empirical research that led to the development and construction of the SSF.

SSF Index Assessment/Treatment Planning

When using CAMS with suicidal patients, the first three pages of the SSF—Sections A–D—are used in the index session when suicidal risk is first identified.

Section A: SSF Likert Ratings

Over a 15-year period the SSF has gone through various changes. But the SSF Likert ratings (shown in Figure 2.1) have remained largely unchanged with only some minor modifications. In this regard, I often refer to this initial section as the "core" SSF assessment section.

The first three SSF Likert assessment constructs (pain, press, and perturbation) are based on the theoretical work of Edwin Shneidman (1988); these items

_____	**1) RATE PSYCHOLOGICAL PAIN** (*hurt, anguish, or misery in your mind; **not** stress; **not** physical pain*): **Low Pain: 1 2 3 4 5 :High Pain** What I find most painful is: _____
_____	**2) RATE STRESS** (*your general feeling of being pressured or overwhelmed*): **Low Stress: 1 2 3 4 5 :High Stress** What I find most stressful is: _____
_____	**3) RATE AGITATION** (*emotional urgency; feeling that you need to take action; **not** irritation; **not** annoyance*): **Low Agitation: 1 2 3 4 5 :High Agitation** I most need to take action when: _____
_____	**4) RATE HOPELESSNESS** (*your expectation that things will not get better no matter what you do*): **Low Hopelessness: 1 2 3 4 5 :High Hopelessness** I am most hopeless about: _____
_____	**5) RATE SELF-HATE** (*your general feeling of disliking yourself; having no self-esteem; having no self-respect*): **Low Self-Hate: 1 2 3 4 5 :High Self-Hate** What I hate most about myself is: _____
N/A	**6) RATE OVERALL RISK OF SUICIDE:** **Extremely Low Risk: 1 2 3 4 5 :Extremely High Risk** **(will <u>not</u> kill self) (will kill self)**

FIGURE 2.1. SSF core Likert assessments.

make up Shneidman's "Cubic Model of Suicide," which is discussed in more detail later. The fourth item—hopelessness—is based on Aaron Beck's work that refers to expectations that things will not get better no matter what one does (Beck, Rush, Shaw, & Emery, 1979). The fifth item, self-hate, is based on the work of Roy Baumeister (1990), who links intolerable perceptions of self to a need for suicidal escape. Finally, the sixth SSF item is a behavioral index pertaining to overall possibility of taking one's life, which is not linked to any particular theorist. Let us now consider each core Likert construct in a bit more depth.

Psychological Pain. Shneidman (1993) has organized an entire meta-psychology of suicide around the central concept of *psychache*—a profound and seemingly unbearable suffering that exists in the mind's eye of the suicidal person. If we mean to help any suicidal person, Shneidman argues, we must understand that a person's psychache is idiosyncratic and particular to that person. Shneidman further asserts that *all* suicides invariably occur when any person's individually determined psychological pain threshold is exceeded. The only way the potential risk of a suicide can be reduced is by finding some way of raising the threshold to pain, thus increasing a patient's capacity to better tolerate the psychache. In addition, we must find ways of removing or ameliorating the root of the psychological pain itself. As I have discussed elsewhere (Jobes & Nelson, 2006), many important authors have seized on variations of Shneidman's notion in their treatment approaches to severe psychological conditions and to suicide (refer to Chiles & Strosahl, 1995; Ellis & Newman, 1996; Joiner, 2005; Linehan, 1993a; Rudd, Joiner, Jobes, & King, 1999; Rudd, Joiner, & Rajab, 2000).

Press (Stress). Beyond his central emphasis on psychological pain, Shneidman (1993) has further emphasized the concept of *press*, which he borrows from the thinking of Henry Murray (1938). Indeed, fundamental to Murray's personality theory called *personology* was an interactive matrix of various psychological needs and presses. For our purposes, this term refers to those largely external (sometimes internal) pressures, stressors, or demands that impinge upon, move, touch, or psychologically affect an individual. These typically include external things such as relational conflicts, job loss, and events that occur in life that create significant distress; alternatively, however, internal stressors such as command hallucinations can be similarly distressful. Presses are intimately linked to overwhelming feelings: the perception that I am overpowered by psychological demands. It should be noted that we have used the more standard term *stress* on the SSF itself because that word is more commonly understood by the typical patient. In this regard, I continue to use the term *stress* in my further descriptions of Shneidman's press construct for sake of clarity.

Perturbation (Agitation). For some, Shneidman's (1993) construct of perturbation is a bit problematic in terms of meaning as it is sometimes confused with psychological pain. Yet Shneidman insists (and I concur) that perturbation is a unique and crucial construct that is distinct and different from psychological pain. Shneidman asserts that perturbation refers to the state of being emotionally upset, disturbed, and disquieted. In his thinking, perturbation includes both cognitive constriction *and* a penchant for self-harm or ill-advised action. Perturbation can be described as the patient's impulsive desire to do *something* to change or alter his or her current unbearable situation. It is an essential psychological *energy* that is the driving force behind suicidal behaviors. It is not uncommon to see patients in a great deal of psychological pain, with perhaps little to no perturbation. But suicides rarely occur without the psychological "oomph" that is needed to overcome our natural thresholds to avoid pain and death (c.f. Joiner's [2005] work about thresholds for pain and avoidance of death, which can transform into a desire for death). Although it is not exactly synonymous, we have used the term *agitation* on the SSF itself in place of *perturbation* because it is more commonly understood by the typical patient (and is similarly used in this text).

The Cubic Model. As I previously mentioned these three preceding constructs are used by Shneidman to form the Cubic Model of Suicide. Within the field it is well known that there are literally dozens of models that have been developed to conceptualize and understand suicide (see Maris, Berman, & Silverman, 2000)—I have even proffered my own (refer to Berman, Jobes, & Silverman, 2006). But of these models, few can compete with the elegant simplicity of Shneidman's Cubic Model of Suicide. The reason that I like this model so much is that the field for too long has been singularly obsessed with delineating empirically based suicide "risk factors." Mind you, it is important to know about suicide risk factors and I do not eschew the worth of knowing about the various psychosocial correlates of suicide, but they only do so much for us from an assessment standpoint.

For example, one of the best known psychological autopsy findings from completed suicides, replicated many times over, is the fact that over 90% of people who kill themselves have a psychiatric diagnosis. In the diagnostic language of DSM—the *Diagnostic and Statistical Manual of Mental Disorders* (American Psychiatric Association, 1994)—we know that the presence of an Axis I or II disorder is highly correlated with the vast majority of completed suicides. What does this important risk factor finding mean in terms of assessment? To wit, my entire caseload has a DSM diagnosis; does that then mean that they are all at risk for suicide? No, not at all.

From another vantage point, I am always trying to reconcile disparities in the suicidal nature of two specific patients that I have seen. One patient I saw at the Veterans Affairs (VA) hospital was diagnosed with schizoaffective disorder. He was routinely tortured by vicious and taunting voices, he was often living on the street, his life was abjectly miserable. Yet, he never ever thought of suicide; in fact, it never even occurred to him as an option. Compare this case to a second patient that I saw in my university's counseling center. She was an outstanding young woman—pretty and intelligent from a seemingly lovely family. Yet, this young patient was plagued with suicidal thoughts and had made three notable overdoses since she was a teenager. My point is that the purely risk factor–driven approach to assessment would place my VA patient at a much higher level of objective risk, whereas my second patient had no business, so to speak, being suicidal at all from a purely risk factor–based perspective.

All this discussion is meant to underscore the singular virtue of Shneidman's Cubic Model of Suicide because it gets us thinking about the suicide risk assessment problem in *three dimensions*. Indeed, the Cubic Model of Suicide helps us think about situation specificity—how does an at-risk person find him- or herself in situations that spark a suicidal act? As shown in Figure 2.2, the Cubic Model of Suicide conceptualizes suicidal behaviors as occurring from a synergy of the three psychological forces that we have just discussed. Each of Shneidman's constructs of pain, press, and perturbation exists on one of three axes in the model and can be rated from low (1) to high (5). Within this model, Shneidman has asserted that *every* suicidal act occurs when maximum levels of psychological pain, stress, and agitation are realized.

The lethal 5–5–5 corner cubelet of the model is particularly noteworthy as a very dangerous intersection and interaction of the three psychological forces. Plainly, the 5–5–5 conceptual corner of this model provides an excellent operational definition of clear and imminent danger to self. Thus the model can obviously be used to directly inform the assessment of suicide risk, but beyond assessment, the model also can be used to formulate and target clinical interventions.

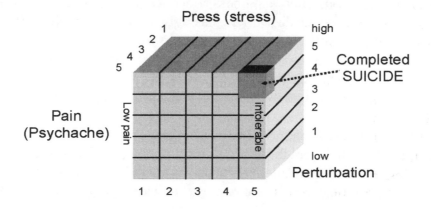

FIGURE 2.2. Shneidman's Cubic Model of Suicide. From Shneidman (1987). Copyright 1987 by the American Psychological Association. Reprinted by permission.

Any clinical intervention that targets any of the three conceptual axes has the potential to meaningfully move a high-risk suicidal patient into a less dangerous psychological space. That means that if one can clinically help reduce psychological pain, or decrease the stressors in the patient's life, or somehow find a way to ameliorate the upset, the potential for suicidal action can be significantly reduced. For example, from my years working with suicidal college students in a counseling center I knew that one of my most powerful interventions involved the engagement of the dean of students who could help deal with faculty such that a student in academic trouble could receive an incomplete or withdrawal from a course without penalty. In reference to the Cubic Model of Suicide, this simple intervention often significantly decreased the academic stress in the student's life, making it more possible to engage the student in psychotherapy, which helped decrease the perturbation, which in turn enabled us to work on the psychosocial causes of the student's psychache.

The Cubic Model of Suicide is therefore the central assessment/treatment hub of the SSF. It provides a three-dimensional assessment window into the patient's suicidal mind that meaningfully eclipses any one-dimensional linear way of thinking about suicide risk assessment. Having now thoroughly argued the virtue of a phenomenological approach to suicide risk, let us shift to three additional theoretical constructs that complete the initial SSF assessment core. These additional constructs help contribute to an even fuller assessment of suicidal risk with direct implications for clinical treatments.

Hopelessness. Aaron Beck's concept of hopelessness refers to one's expectation that a negative situation will not get better no matter what one does to change that situation. Hopelessness is intimately linked to future thinking and represents a third leg of Beck's larger theory of depression that emphasizes the cognitive triad—a sense of hopelessness about self, others, and the future. Future thinking as it relates to suicide is an increasingly important construct that is being more widely discussed in the suicidology literature (e.g., Williams, 2001). As the founder of cognitive therapy, Beck has led the way in our evolving appreciation of the critical role that *thinking* plays in various psychological and psychiatric problems. While Beck is widely known for his pioneering work in the development of cognitive therapy for the treatment of depression, his contributions to suicide prevention are quite notable. Indeed, Beck was the 1983 recipient of the Louis I. Dublin Award from the AAS in recognition of career contributions to the field of suicide prevention. In my own view, Beck's theoretical and empirical work in the area of *hopelessness* as it relates to suicide is a particularly noteworthy contribution (Beck et al., 1979).

Within our own research group we have unpublished data that shows distinctly different cognitive content for college students ($n = 201$) who are suicidal versus college students (n = 201) who are not suicidal (Nademin, Jobes, Downing, & Mann, 2005). In terms of future thinking, we found that our nonsuicidal sample had over *twice* as much self-reported *plans and goals* and *hopes for the future* than our suicidal sample. In addition, we found our nonsuicidal sample had significantly more *belief*-based reasons for living. It is clear that the capacity to think about the future with a sense of hope is absolutely protective against suicide. It follows that a sense of hopefulness within our future thinking and key beliefs help us weather the rough spots that we invariably encounter in life. Alternatively, the absence of hopefulness—particularly in the absolute sense of hopelessness—is an extremely pernicious risk factor for suicide. Indeed, in terms of prospective research there is perhaps no single construct that has been more highly correlated with completed suicide than hopelessness (Beck, 1986; Brown, Beck, Steer, & Grisham, 2000).

Given this discussion, I felt it was imperative to include hopelessness as a key SSF construct. For starters, it has both theoretical and empirical support, but there is also a clinically relevant aspect related to actively working with the construct of *hope*. While the relative presence or absence of hope is extremely important to note from an assessment standpoint, it also provides an organizing focus for treatment. For example, it is a good idea to develop a line of psychotherapy that specifically targets the importance of future thinking and overtly emphasizes the need to build a sense of hope. I remember an early supervisor of mine insisting that we must be "hope vendors" to our patients. This notion strikes me as being uniformly true and central to successful treatment in general and particularly true when working with suicidal people.

Self-Regard (Self-Hate). There are many psychodynamic and psychoanalytic approaches to suicide (refer to a more thorough discussion of theory in Berman et al., 2006) and I felt compelled to include a construct on the SSF that captured some of this valuable thinking. Generically speaking, these theories tend to emphasize unconscious aspects of suicide, interpersonal aspects of suicide, and notions related to killing off the self. Ultimately, an approach that most captured different thinking along these lines was developed by Roy Baumeister (who actually is not a psychodynamic theorist). Baumeister's (1990) paper conceptualizing suicide as an escape from self is a classic; in his view suicidal people are fundamentally driven to psychologically escape unacceptable perceptions of self. According to Baumeister's theory, one's negative views of the self can become so unbearable (i.e., one's self-loathing and self-hatred is so extreme) that suicide becomes a compelling means to escape this intolerable perception of self. Bottom line, there is an intense psychological need to escape.

In this regard, we have a great deal of empirical data that underscores the intensity of this need for escape in suicidal people (Jobes, 2005; Jobes & Mann,

1999). In research studies that we have conducted with suicidal college students and active duty Air Force personnel, we have found that the need for escape is cited by these patients as a major reason for wanting to die. In fact among our Air Force sample, over 60% of our Reasons for Dying responses were variations on themes of escape (Jobes, 2004b).

Beyond escape, Baumeister's approach emphasizes the self. From Carl Jung to Heinz Kohut, the notion of self is a central construct within psychodynamically oriented metapsychology. Intuitively we know that people who think about suicide are fundamentally preoccupied with their unhappiness, in most cases that misery is often psychologically rooted close to home—in the person's sense of self. It is perhaps self-evident that people who love themselves or are fundamentally comfortable with who they are most likely are not inclined to take their lives. In many respects successful psychotherapy often centers on a systematic deconstruction followed by a subsequent reconstruction of the patient's sense of self. Thus, the beauty of Baumeister's conceptual approach is that it captures two essential components of the suicidal struggle—the need for escape and the core importance of the self.

Behavioral Assessment of Suicidal Risk. Finally, there was a need to capture the bottom-line *behavioral* possibility of suicide on the SSF (i.e., is this person going to actually take his or her own life?). This final assessment construct does not cite any particular theorist but obviously captures in a generic sense the behavioral perspective on suicide risk. In this regard, the sixth Likert scale on the SSF simply asks whether or not the patient will or will not kill him- or herself. This question is not only significant because of the obvious implications for life and death but also because it goes to one of the most essential and elusive struggles in clinical suicidology—namely, the medicolegal challenge to determine whether there is a "clear and imminent" risk for suicidal behavior. Let us consider for a moment the issue of risk from a legal standpoint. What exactly does "clear and imminent" danger to self mean? In my experience, suicidal states are hardly ever "clear." Invariably suicidal states are much more shades of gray rather than crystal. And what about "imminent"? Does it mean, right this second, later today, or sometime this week? While exact definitions of these terms are elusive, these terms are important for the safety of the patient and have significant implications for the potential liability of the clinician if a suicide occurs. Given all these considerations, it obviously made sense to include a behavioral assessment of risk as a final Likert construct on the SSF.

Psychometrics of SSF Likert Ratings

There are solid empirical data in support of the validity and reliability of the core SSF Likert ratings (Jobes, Jacoby, Cimbolic, & Hustead, 1997). The 1997 study was conducted with a sample of suicidal college students (n = 103) and used sub-samples of nonclinical college students (Jobes et al., 1997). In this study we established that the six core SSF Likert constructs function quasi-independently from each other (i.e., there was no between variable multicolinearity). The SSF variables also demonstrated statistically significant convergent and criterion-prediction validity. Finally, test–retest reliability of the SSF variables was statistically significant with good to excellent with reliability coefficients ranging from .3 to .7. Even though the psychometrics of the SSF are quite good, we continue to try to improve the tool. At the time of this writing, a major psychometric replication study is under way with a large inpatient sample of adult suicide attempters and ideators at the Mayo Clinic in Rochester, Minnesota (Lineberry et al., 2006). This study should help further clarify the psychometrics of the SSF with a more severe population, which will further improve the internal validity and generalizability of the core SSF Likert assessment constructs.

Qualitative SSF Assessments

One of the most notable features of the SSF is the inclusion of various qualitative assessments. As I have discussed elsewhere (Jobes et al., 2004), the addition of qualitative assessments to the previously discussed quantitative assessments is a novel idea because most psychological assessment tools are either quantitative *or* qualitative (narrative); these two entirely different approaches are rarely integrated within the same assessment tool. It is my strong contention that each type of assessment approach has much to offer individually, but taken together using both quantitative and qualitative provides a much fuller picture of virtually any suicidal state. Embedded within the SSF are three different qualitative assessments: (1) the SSF qualitative Likert prompts, (2) the SSF Reasons for Living versus Reasons for Dying assessment, and (3) the SSF One-Thing Response. Each of these assessments is discussed here in more depth related to empirical research as well as clinical assessment and treatment implications.

SSF Qualitative Likert Prompts. Recent research on the SSF qualitative Likert prompts has provided valuable insights about the nature and content of suicidal thoughts among those who seek mental health care (Jobes et al., 1997). This particular SSF assessment is akin to Rotter's (Rotter & Rafferty, 1950) projective assessment, the Incomplete Sentence Blank (ISB). The idea is that the five sentence stems prompt an opportunity for the patient to respond *in his or her own written words*. As shown in Figure 2.1, each of the five SSF qualitative stems are followed by a 5-inch line of space for the patient to hand write a response. For example, in relation to the psychological pain question, suicidal patients who are completing the SSF provide a response to "What I find most painful is. . . ." As discussed further in Chapter 3, the clinician encourages the patient to respond to each of the

SSF sentence stems, as the patient writes in his or her own hand what comes to mind in reaction to each SSF incomplete sentence.

As shown in Appendix B, a coding manual was carefully developed through a modified consensual validation process (Jobes et al., 2004). The coding manual was developed through a rigorous five-step methodology—two naive coders were trained to use the coding system and were able to sort all written responses into content categories (see Table 2.1) with very high interrater reliability (kappas > .80).

This coding manual was used to examine the SSF qualitative Likert prompts from two different samples of suicidal outpatients seeking treatment. The first sample included suicidal college students (n = 119). The second sample included active-duty U.S. Air Force personnel (n = 33). These two distinctly different samples provided a wide range of 636 written responses to the five SSF prompts. Not surprisingly, certain written qualitative responses of these patients were more frequent than others, both within and across the five SSF constructs. Among a range of specific exploratory findings, one general finding was that two-thirds of the 636 obtained written responses could be reliably categorized (refer back to Table 2.1) under four major content headings: *Relational* (22%), *Role Responsibilities* (20%), *Self* (15%), and *Unpleasant Internal States* (10%). To my knowledge, I am not aware of any other study that has so specifically accessed and investigated the content of suicidal thinking.

To be honest, prior to conducting the study, I would have expected many more responses coded under the Unpleasant Internal States coding category (e.g., expressions of depression, anxiety, misery, and despair) because there is so much emphasis in the suicidology literature on psychopathology. Instead what we saw was a predominance of responses linked to relational and vocational issues. Perhaps Sigmund Freud was right when he argued that happiness in life centers on *work* and *love* (Gay, 1989). Our third most frequent type of responses related to issues of self. As discussed earlier, self-related issues are a focal construct in psychodynamic thinking; indeed, beyond psychodynamic theory one could argue that the notion of self is central within our larger Western metapsychology.

Intrapsychic versus Interpsychic Suicide Risk Assessment. As I discussed in a 1995 paper (Jobes, 1995a), data from our research shows that some suicidal patients are psychologically very internally focused in their suicidality. In cases of "intrapsychic" suicidality, the thoughts of the suicidal person are kept private and suicides occur as a surprise to others. These suicidal states are thought to be more associated with major psychiatric disorders—DSM major psychiatric Axis I disorders (e.g., major depression). In contrast, "interpsychically" suicidal people are those whose suicidal thoughts are diectly related to relational issues; others routinely know about their suicidal thoughts and

TABLE 2.1. Definitions of Coding Categories and Example Responses

Category	Definition	Examples
1. Relational[a]	Any references to specific relationship problems or issues with family, friends, or significant others or any other social interaction. Any responses that speak to being hurt by others, hurting others, or being alone and isolated go here as well.	"Loss of my father." "Loneliness."
2. Self[b]	Responses that are specific to one's self, or when a reference to one's self is clearly inferred. These can be statements about feelings or qualities about the self. These tend to be descriptors of core attributes or harsh self-critiques of external descriptors.	"I hate myself." "I'm a bad person."
3. Helpless[c]	Any implied or specific references to feeling out of control, lost, trapped, or directionless. Includes statements about hopelessness about one's ability to cope, function, or achieve in the future.	"Being out of control." "There's no way out."
4. Global/ General[a]	Any nonspecific, broad statements that are completely inclusive and therefore vague. These responses indicate a general overarching sense of being overwhelmed and/or unable to cope.	"Everything." "Overwhelm-ingness."
5. Unpleasant Internal States[b]	Statements referring to specific, discrete descriptions of hurting, distress, suffering, pain, and other negative emotions.	"Anxiety." "Hurting and misery."
6. Unsure/ Unable to Articulate[a]	Statements in which the person is uncertain/unable to respond. May include responses that seem purposely evasive, avoidant, or apathetic.	"Unsure." "I don't know."
7. Role Responsi-bilities[a]	Common adult role expectations including the roles of the worker, homemaker, or student. Responses such as academic concerns, financial burdens, or job concerns are included here. Specific future-oriented statements regarding career are also included.	"I'm a bad parent." "Failing this class."
8. Situation Specific[d]	Any reference made about a specific situation or circumstance, or any references made to a certain place, time, or events.	"When I awake." "Coming home alone."
9. Compelled to Act[e]	Explicit desire to urgently change one's life; a quick solution; a need to take action; being stuck.	"This needs to end." "I can't take it anymore."

(continued)

TABLE 2.1. *(continued)*

Category	Definition	Examples
10. Future[f]	Specific dreams, skills, events, or experiences (except career or school, see Role/Responsibilities) with a clear reference to the future.	"My future." "Achieving my dreams."
11. Internal Descriptors[g]	Lack of positive qualities or the presence of negative qualities in him-/herself; feelings about the self; inner descriptors of the self.	"I'm a coward." "I'm an idiot."
12. External Descriptors[g]	Some external, outer aspect of him/herself such as his/her personal appearance, body, or behaviors in which he/she is engaging.	"I'm fat." "My drug use."

[a] Applies to pain, press, perturbation, hopelessness, and self-hate.
[b] Applies to pain, press, perturbation, and hopelessness.
[c] Applies to pain, press, perturbation, and self-hate.
[d] Applies to press and perturbation.
[e] Applies to perturbation only.
[f] Applies to hopelessness only.
[g] Applies to self-hate only.

threats and suicidal acts are precipitated by interpersonal events. These suicidal states are more associated with personality disorders—DSM Axis II disorders. Other research and theory have largely supported this approach and are discussed further on (Fazaa & Page, 2003, 2005).

SSF Reasons for Living (RFL) versus Reasons for Dying (RFD). As shown in Figure 2.3, the next qualitative SSF assessment involves an examination of the suicidal patient's reasons for wanting to live versus reasons for wanting to die (RFL vs. RFD).

Rank	REASONS FOR LIVING	Rank	REASONS FOR DYING

FIGURE 2.3. SSF Reasons for Living versus Reasons for Dying.

In my experience of talking to suicidal patients over the past 20 years, I have been struck by the internal debate inherent in the suicidal struggle. On the one hand, most of these patients have many thoughts about why they want to die; while on the other hand, these same patients invariably have at least one or two reasons (or more) for still wanting to live. Now it is important to keep in mind that both my clinical experience and our empirical data are from suicidal people who are seeking mental health care. I would therefore speculate that those suicidal people who do not seek mental health care may be perhaps somewhat less ambivalent because they are not with someone who is charged with stopping the suicidal act. We do know from psychological autopsy studies that suicidal patients are commonly ambivalent; they may still be struggling with the decision of choosing death over life right up to the moment of their death. Accordingly, this ambivalence is the cornerstone to clinical success with suicidal patients; we must capitalize on that sense of uncertainty and fight on behalf of that side that harbors thoughts of life, which dares to want to live even in the face of abject pain and suffering.

Our qualitative research on RFL versus RFD (Jobes & Mann, 1999, 2000) was built on the important work of Marsha Linehan, the developer of the Reasons for Living Inventory (Linehan, Goodstein, Nielson, & Chiles, 1983). Linehan had the novel idea of studying suicide risk assessment in an entirely different way. With dozens of studies dedicated to risk factors and why people might want to die, Linehan argued that an equally compelling assessment notion was the value of examining why any person might want to live. In effect, the absence of RFL could be inversely correlated to increased suicide risk. Building on this line of thinking we have argued that there is actually tremendous value in considering both sides of the life-versus-death coin, *simultaneously* in the same assessment (Jobes & Mann, 2000)

To illustrate, I once had a case of a compelling patient who was highly suicidal. When I asked him to complete the SSF RFL versus RFD assessment, he had no problem quickly writing down 5 reasons for wanting to die and then added another 5 reasons just as readily—10 reasons for dying! I gently urged him to provide some RFL and he consequently broke down in tears. No need for a discriminant function analysis in this case—this was clearly a highly suicidal person. When I gently pushed for any reason to live, he eventually mentioned his beloved dog. All this was very interesting considering that he had earlier reported to me that he was married to a "wonderful" woman. When I pointed out this observation, he noted that he partitioned his depression and suicidal suffering away from his wife; she had no idea how deadly serious his depression had become. Indeed, in this case the patient argued that taking his life would be doing his wife a favor—this idea of "perceived burdensomeness" is commonly seen among suicidal people (Joiner, 2005).

One particularly compelling aspect of these qualitative SSF responses goes beyond mere assessment considerations. Referring to the previous case example, it was immediately clear that couple therapy was urgently in order. In turn, when the couple subsequently met with me, the patient was actually genuinely surprised when his horrified wife made it quite plain that she would in fact *not* be better off without him! In fact, she argued quite convincingly that his potential suicide would burden her with an irreversible legacy of regret and loss that would haunt her for the rest of her life. Thus, this simple assessment led to a powerful reason for wanting to live—to not let down his wife. Bottom line in terms of treatment implications, a fairly simple idea emerges: For treatment to work with suicidal patients, both the clinician and patient must set about systematically eliminating reasons for dying while simultaneously working to develop, infuse, and increase more reasons for wanting to live. Our research (Jobes & Mann, 1999; Mann, 2002) has shown that we can reliably code various RFL versus RFD responses under the category headings shown in Table 2.2, which depicts data obtained from 201 suicidal college students seeking counseling center mental health care (Mann, 2002).

As we can see in this table, suicidal patients provide a number of striking RFL responses. These coding categories of responses are intuitive and capture what, for most of us, makes the world go round. In fact, we have found in a large sample of nonsuicidal college students (n = 201) that these various RFL categories capture the responses of a nonclinical sample very well (Jobes, 2004b; Nademin et al., 2005).

In the Nademin and colleagues (2005) study, we set about comparing exclusively the RFL responses of this non-suicidal sample to a large sample (n = 201) of suicidal patients who had sought treatment at university counseling centers (Mann, 2002). As shown in Table 2.3, there were some strikingly significant differences among the responses of these two groups. Specifically, the suicidal sample had significantly more responses that focus on family and a desire not to burden loved ones with their suicide (interestingly, this is the opposite of Joiner's notion related to perceived burdensomeness). Moreover, the suicidal group cited significantly more RFL pertaining to a desire for enjoyable things (e.g., listening to music or enjoying *The Simpsons*—the long-running cartoon TV show). In contrast, the nonsuicidal sample of students had significantly more plans and goals, hopes for the future, and beliefs.

My interpretation of these RFL data speaks to a *loss/deficit orientation* of suicidal patients, in contrast to *gain/surplus orientation* of the nonsuicidal sample. For instance, note that overall in terms of sheer frequencies of RFL responses, the nonsuicidal sample has almost twice as many responses (frequency = 1,004) than the suicidal sample does (frequency = 598). To clarify, the suicidal sample that completed the RFL versus RFD section of the SSF were not required to fill in all

TABLE 2.2. Frequencies of Responses in Each Category for Reasons for Living and Reasons for Dying

Category	Frequency	Percentage
Reasons for Living		
Plans and Goals	108	18.1
Family	99	16.6
Enjoyable Things	88	14.7
Hopefulness for the Future	76	12.7
Friends	61	10.2
Self	58	9.7
Burdening Others	49	8.2
Beliefs	34	5.7
Responsibility to Others	25	4.2
Reasons for Dying		
General Descriptors of Self	160	31.1
Escape in General	125	24.3
Others/Relationships	57	11.1
Escape Pain	54	10.5
Hopelessness	52	10.1
Unburdening Others	22	4.3
Escape Responsibilities	21	4.1
Loneliness	20	3.9
Escape Past	3	0.6

Note. Total number of RFL responses = 598; total number of RFD responses = 514

the spaces—the majority neither gave us five reasons for wanting to live nor gave us five reasons for wanting to die. The nonsuicidal sample that were recruited from introductory psychology courses were similarly not instructed to fill in all five RFL spaces, yet clearly many of them did. On the one hand, the striking differences in frequencies could be an artifact of the situation—motivation to fully complete all spaces may have been induced in a course-credit scenario, which is obviously different than a clinical situation. On the other hand, however, perhaps these nonsuicidal students just have a lot more reasons for which they want to live. Such a simplistic interpretation of these data must be viewed with caution, but such an interpretation does seem reasonable. Whatever the case, in comparison to the suicidal sample, the nonsuicidal sample clearly had a surplus of RFL that were *aspirational*—gain-oriented in nature.

The loss-oriented suicidal sample was motivated to live because of the perceived impact their suicide would have on others. In addition, the suicidal sample

TABLE 2.3. Reasons for Living: Nonsuicidal versus Suicidal Samples

Reasons for living	Nonclinical sample ($n = 201$)		Clinical sample ($n - 201$)		Chi-square
	Frequency	Percentage	Frequency	Percentage	
Family	89	8.86	99	16.6	22.16*
Friends	86	8.57	61	10.2	1.36
Responsibility to Others	45	4.48	25	4.2	0.06
Burdening Others	12	1.2	49	8.2	50.84*
Plans and Goals	312	31.08	108	18.1	31.41*
Hopefulness for the Future	241	24.00	76	12.7	29.02*
Enjoyable Things	28	2.79	88	14.7	80.61*
Beliefs	90	8.96	34	5.7	5.37*
Self	101	10.06	58	9.7	0.03
Total	1,004		598		

Note. Data from Nademin, Jobes, Downing, and Mann (2005).
*$p < .05$.

was preoccupied with the loss of things they actually enjoy such as good food, music, certain TV shows, and the like. In sharp contrast, the gain or surplus-oriented nonsuicidal sample is preoccupied with various plans, goals, hopes for the future, and beliefs. This group clearly has a forward-thinking orientation to life with uplifting goals to which they aspire.

Consequently, the assessment implications of these data are significant and the treatment implications are notable. If one sees a suicidal patient with limited or no plans, hopes, goals for the future, or beliefs, then treatment must include developing these uplifting aspirational goals. It is my sense that anyone can get through a rough patch if they have hope and a belief that things will one day change and improve. In contrast, we know that suicidal people have fundamental and critical deficits in the areas of looking forward with hope and sustaining such aspiring beliefs.

SSF Wish to Live versus Wish to Die Assessment. Maria Kovacs and Aaron Beck (1977) wrote an important paper arguing for an "internal struggle hypothesis"—that suicidal people struggle through between competing wishes for living versus dying. This is a similar notion to the preceding discussion of reasons for living versus dying and seemed like a worthwhile brief assessment to include on the SSF for both clinical and research purposes.

SSF One-Thing Response. Similar to the preceding qualitative assessments, the SSF One-Thing Response gathers useful information directly from patients about the one thing that would make them no longer suicidal. In our research we have seen a remarkable range of responses to this question (Jobes, 2004b). For example, one suicidal Air Force patient in one of our studies wrote: "five million dollars and a ticket home." Frankly this response is rather flip and not particularly useful clinically. In contrast, however, I once had a patient write: "to get my medications right—I have been having mood swings related to mixing my oral contraceptive with my anti-depressant medicine." Such a response is much more clinically helpful, prompting an immediate referral to a consulting psychiatrist. In comparing these two examples I do not mean to be pejorative about the first example, it is just that the second example provides the clinician with much more useful clinical information that leads directly to a treatment intervention.

Recent unpublished research (Fratto, Jobes, Pentiuc, Rice, & Tendick, 2004) has shown that a reliable coding system has been developed that can organize these responses within three domains: (1) self versus other-oriented responses, (2) realistic versus unrealistic responses, and (3) clinically useful versus clinically not useful responses. With a relatively large sample ($n = 191$) of suicidal college students seeking treatment at a university counseling center, we found that those SSF One-Thing Responses that were self-oriented, realistic, and clinically useful had significantly better categorical treatment outcomes than other permutations of other One-Thing Responses. This may be an obvious finding, but neverthe-less our data show that it is very important that clinicians take note of these responses in the index session as they may have implications for treatment and outcomes.

Section B: SSF Empirically Based Risk Variables

As shown in Figure 2.4, the SSF empirically based risk variables that appear on the second page of the index SSF assessment (Section B) are well-researched, empirically based risk factors that are among the best variables for suicide risk (Joiner, Walker, Rudd, & Jobes, 1999; Oordt, Jobes, et al., 2005).

Although there are literally dozens of potential psychosocial risk factor correlates for attempted and completed suicidal behavior, this particular set of variables was partly derived with help by a work group of experts convened by the U.S. Air Force Suicide Prevention Program (refer to Oordt, Jobes, et al., 2005, for more discussion of this work group). These variables have been used in early SSF versions and have proven to be a valuable short list of suicide risk variables with good empirical support (Berman et al., 2006; Jobes & Berman, 1993; Jobes et al., 1997).

Section B (*Clinician*):

Y N Suicide Plan:	When: _____	
	Where: _____	
	How: _____	Y N Access to means
	How: _____	Y N Access to means
Y N Suicide Preparation	Describe: _____	
Y N Suicide Rehearsal	Describe: _____	
Y N History of Suicidality		
• Ideation	Describe: _____	
• Frequency	_____ per day _____ per week _____ per month	
• Duration	_____ seconds _____ minutes _____ hours	
• Single Attempt	Describe: _____	
• Multiple Attempts	Describe: _____	
Y N Current Intent	Describe: _____	
Y N Impulsivity	Describe: _____	
Y N Substance Abuse	Describe: _____	
Y N Significant Loss	Describe: _____	
Y N Interpersonal Isolation	Describe: _____	
Y N Relationship Problems	Describe: _____	
Y N Health Problems	Describe: _____	
Y N Physical Pain	Describe: _____	
Y N Legal Problems	Describe: _____	
Y N Shame	Describe: _____	

FIGURE 2.4. SSF empirically based risk variables.

Section C: SSF Treatment Planning

Section C of the SSF (see Figure 2.5) is a treatment planning section that is discussed in depth in Chapter 5. Suffice it to say, this section is unique in that the treatment plan directly flows from the collaborative assessment performed by the patient and clinician in Sections A and B. For our current consideration, there are a few points to emphasize about Section C.

To begin with, unlike traditional treatment planning where the clinician alone writes up the patient's plan (and may or may not share that plan with the patient), the CAMS approach emphasizes collaborative treatment planning in which the patient functions as a *coauthor* of the plan (Jobes & Drozd, 2004). The premise is that the clinician is now uniquely positioned to consider various interventions *with* the patient having collaboratively completed SSF assessment Sections A and B. Within the CAMS approach, a central and overt goal is to consider what interventions will be necessary to be able to justify *outpatient* care. In other words, collaboratively developing an outpatient treatment plan is an overarching goal of CAMS. Accordingly, it is important to note that within the SSF treatment planning section there is a preexisting number-one clinical problem—"Self-Harm Potential." In turn, this primary clinical problem focus leads to a preexisting clinical goal/objective—"Outpatient Safety." This particular clinical problem and goal is then followed by spaces for "Interventions" and the "Estimated # of Sessions." This sequence of treatment planning considerations is important because the number-one clinical problem is frankly not negotiable. If the clinician and patient are not able to sufficiently address the clinical problem of self-harm potential through their collaborative treatment planning, an inpatient hospitalization may be necessary as the only means of ensuring the patient's immediate physical safety.

Following this line of thinking, there is a need for the clinician and patient to seriously consider how they can develop a time-specific plan to best ensure the patient's outpatient stability and safety. In this regard, CAMS emphasizes the development and use of a "Crisis Response Plan," which is a relatively new and alternative approach to the use of "safety contracts" or "no-suicide contracts." As discussed by Rudd, Joiner, and Rajab (2001), the Crisis Response Plan emphasizes what a patient prospectively *will* do should they become acutely depressed, impulsive, and suicidal. In other words, specific actions and interventions are clearly planned in anticipation of potential crises. In contrast, outpatient safety contracting as it is typically used tends to emphasize what patients *will not* do through a *promise* that they will not hurt themselves. As this safety contract approach is often used, there is usually no consideration of what the patient should do (instead of self-harm behavior) should a crisis occur.

In summary, there is a clear emphasis in CAMS on outpatient treatment planning—using a time-specific Crisis Response Plan approach—that is collaboratively drafted by the clinician and patient *together*. There will be a much more detailed discussion of CAMS outpatient treatment planning and use of the Crisis Response Plan in Chapter 5.

Problem #	Problem Description	Goals and Objectives Evidence for Attainment	Interventions (Type and Frequency)	Estimated # Sessions
1	Self-Harm Potential	Outpatient Safety	Crisis Response Plan:	
2				
3				

FIGURE 2.5. SSF Outpatient Treatment Planning.

Section D: SSF HIPAA Forms

During the 1990s, the U.S Congress passed a significant piece of legislation with profound implications for health care delivery. The Health Insurance Portability and Accountability Act (HIPAA) was passed (in part) as a means of ensuring the privacy and security of medical health records as well as standardizing practices related to personal health information (e.g., rules related to electronic transmission). The legislation required full compliance of providers across health care disciplines as of April 13, 2003. The implications of HIPAA have been far-reaching for all health care providers, including mental health professionals. Incorporating key elements of HIPAA into the SSF was obvious considering the overall importance of HIPAA and its clear emphasis on standardizing and improving the quality of medical records.

Therefore at each phase within CAMS—Index Assessment/Treatment Planning, Clinical Tracking, and Clinical Outcomes—there are specific pages that are referred to as the "HIPAA pages" of the SSF (pages 3, 5, and 7 of the SSF as shown in Appendix A). The inclusion of these particular pages is meant to provide an efficient way of maintaining a medical record that complies with criteria under the provisions of HIPAA. As discussed in Chapter 8, the protective aspects of careful documentation in relation to malpractice litigation is important to appreciate. In relation to these various considerations, the SSF has been specifically constructed to be protective from a liability perspective *and* be fully compliant with HIPAA-related provisions.

As an important point of reference, when CAMS was used in Air Force outpatient clinics, the various pages of the SSF served as *the* medical record for suicidal outpatients while on Suicide Status. In other words, while suicidal patients were being tracked using the SSF there was no replication of mental health care information elsewhere in the chart. When resolution of Suicide Status is achieved, the clinician can transition back to the medical records that are routinely used.

This emphasis on well-documented assessment and treatment is important for a number of reasons. For example, according to the Joint Commission on Accreditation of Healthcare Organizations (JCAHO)—the central organizing body that accredits hospitals throughout the United States—the number-one sentinel event (failure in medical care leading to fatalities) for the last number of years has been failures linked to suicides. JCAHO has thus pushed hard for hospitals and accredited facilities to do a better job of documenting their assessment and treatment of suicidal risk. At one of the Air Force Life Skills Clinics in Colorado that used CAMS with suicidal patients, this approach and the related quality of medical record was cited by JCAHO inspectors as a "best practice."

Use of the SSF in a variety of settings (e.g., outpatient clinics, hospitals, and hotline crisis centers) has made me aware of the need for some adaptations depending on the setting. For example, certain university counseling centers have opted not to use the "HIPAA" pages of the SSF, arguing that the nature of work in these centers does not meet the criteria for being HIPAA compliant. In these settings, only four SSF pages (pages 1, 2, 4, and 6 as seen in Appendix A) are used. I have been open to this modified use of the SSF, in recognition that counseling centers have historically used a more developmental approach to care with less emphasis on diagnosis and psychopathology. Although I still generally recommend the use of all of the pages of the SSF to ensure maximal documentation (which reduces vulnerability to liability), I do recognize the need for adaptations and alternative uses depending on the setting.

SSF Tracking Forms

Another innovative element of CAMS and the SSF is the use of SSF Tracking Forms that administratively "track" a suicidal patient. As used in CAMS, the administration of the first three pages of SSF in the index session is not a singular event but the beginning of an ongoing process within CAMS (for patients who are then considered to be on Suicide Status). This process includes clinical assessment, treatment, and modification of treatment until outcomes occur. As I discuss in much greater detail in Chapter 6, the ongoing assessment of suicidal risk in a Suicide Status patient involves a series of SSF follow-up assessments that mark the beginning of each clinical session. Within CAMS, the topic of suicide does not "fall through the cracks"—it is directly addressed at the start of every session for the duration of time that the patient remains on Suicide Status. Moreover, the suicide specific treatment plan within CAMS is monitored and changed as needed, with the goal of systematically eliminating the option of suicide as a means of coping with seemingly unbearable pain and suffering.

SSF Resolution Forms

When the suicidal risk is clinically resolved over the course of care, the appropriate SSF resolution forms (pages 6 and 7—see Appendix A) are completed and the patient is no longer considered to be on Suicide Status (see Chapter 7 for a detailed discussion of how CAMS resolution and outcomes are determined). These forms are crucial in terms of providing documentation of clinical outcomes within the CAMS framework. They also provide a meaningful marker of clinical progress as the clinician and patient demarcate the resolution of the suicidal risk that was first identified and assessed in the index session.

THE ORIGIN OF CAMS

Now that we have a sense of the SSF, it is worth noting how a particular application of the SSF led to the origin of the CAMS approach. Over the first 10 years of SSF research and clinical use, the form was *not* completed collaboratively. Originally, the core SSF Likert section was completed by both the clinician and the patient independently of each other at the end of the index session. The original thinking was that having independent ratings of these constructs might prove clinically useful in order to catch certain discrepancies between the respective sets of ratings. To that end, we did in fact observe some statistically significant differences between clinician and patient ratings (Jobes et al., 1997). Overall, however, the clinician and patient ratings were typically more similar than different.

The idea of collaboratively completing the SSF was born out of an initiative to further develop the use of the SSF in a large outpatient managed mental health care system. Our first efforts to use the SSF in a collaborative fashion was very well received by clinicians and patients alike, particularly when the idea of building collaborative suicide-specific treatment planning section, was layered into a later version of the SSF. Using the feedback of clinicians and their patients, this collaborative use of the SSF marked the genesis of what became the larger CAMS approach described in this book (Jobes, Luoma, Jacoby, & Mann, 1999).

As discussed in the final chapter (Chapter 9), CAMS is now being systematically used in a variety of clinical settings and many individual practitioners whom I have trained are using CAMS with reportedly great success. Along with various collaborators I am currently pursuing further grant funding to conduct a variety of prospective randomized clinical trial studies of CAMS. Clinical studies to date are extremely encouraging in support of using CAMS as a practicable approach to assessing and managing suicidal risk (e.g., Jobes, Wong, Conrad, Drozd, & Neal-Walden, 2005; Kahn-Green, Jobes, Goeke-Morey, & Greene, 2006). Our initial studies of CAMS have used either retrospective or concurrent methodologies that provide correlational data. While these data are extremely encouraging, the definitive "gold standard" test of CAMS awaits the prospective clinical trial studies that are now being developed and pursued.

Initial CAMS Research: A "Real-World" Application

One initial study of CAMS was conducted retrospectively with a sample of suicidal Air Force personnel ($n = 55$) who sought mental health treatment at two U.S. Air Force Life Skills Clinics in Colorado (Jobes et al., 2005). This particular study was a naturalistic examination of a "real-world" application of CAMS that underscores the use of CAMS to address significant clinical challenges and needs (see also Drozd, Jobes, & Luoma, 2000).

At the time we began our research in two "Life Skills" treatment centers at two different Air Force facilities, fully one-third of the patients who routinely sought mental health care had some degree of suicidal ideation. In this situation it was clear that the commanding officers of these outpatient teams did not want any patients taking their lives, but clinical options for such patients were limited particularly as base hospitals no longer had any psychiatric beds. Although there were available beds at nearby private psychiatric hospitals, the lengths of stay were very short and the coordination of care was inconsistent or nonexistent. The young clinicians working in these clinics were both overwhelmed and uncertain about how to treat this significant number of suicidal patients.

After extensive discussions with key collaborators, and some long-distance training over the phone and by e-mail, CAMS was slowly introduced and tried by various clinicians in these outpatient clinics. Over the months that followed the initial use of CAMS, I began to receive enthusiastic e-mails and calls from clinicians in these clinics who felt that they now had an effective new way to work with these challenging suicidal cases. Importantly (from a research standpoint), some clinicians in these settings were enthused about using CAMS, whereas some remained uninterested and declined to use CAMS. This scenario created a naturalistic opportunity to conduct a retrospective (ex post facto) study of CAMS—comparing an "experimental" group (n = 25 cases of suicidal patients seeing clinicians who used CAMS) to a "control" group (n = 30 cases of suicidal patients seeing clinicians who provided "treatment as usual" [TAU]). Obviously there was no random assignment to condition or checks of clinician fidelity as to what was then an early version of CAMS. Thus, experimental internal validity was clearly compromised. However, given the real-world naturalistic use of CAMS in this situation, the external validity was extremely high.

The results of this naturalistic archival study were notable. For example, the suicidal patients in the CAMS treatment group (n = 25) resolved their suicidal ideation in significantly fewer sessions (M =7.35, SD = 4.21) than those in the TAU group (M = 11.4, SD = 7.02), t (35) = 2.08, p = .045, d = .69. This significant effect is visually illustrated by Figure 2.6, which shows the results of a survival analysis conducted on these data. Of 100% of patients in both groups who resolved their suicidal ideation, the CAMS group achieved this goal more quickly, in both a statistically significant and clinically meaningful way.

As can be seen in Figure 2.6, most CAMS patients resolved their ideation within 10 to 12 sessions whereas the TAU group took almost 20 or more sessions to achieve the same effect. Effectively this means that the clinical window of risk for CAMS patients got closed about 4 weeks sooner than it did for patients in the TAU condition. In other words, the CAMS patients much more rapidly extinguished their suicidal thoughts, enabling their clinicians to move onto other treat-

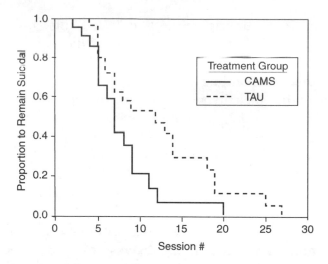

FIGURE 2.6. Survival analysis of CAMS versus TAU.

ment issues with the looming threat of suicidality effectively taken off the thera-peutic table.

As shown in Figure 2.7, there was another set of significant findings that we had not anticipated. Because detailed medical records are maintained on com-puter databases in the military, we were able to observe that, in contrast to the TAU patients, CAMS patients had significantly fewer non-mental health medical appointments in the six months following the suicidal crisis that brought them into the life skills center. Figure 2.7 therefore depicts an interrupted time series analysis of data for patients in both conditions in terms of their medical utiliza-tion (black bars) and their mental health utilization (white bars) for the 6 months prior to the suicidal crisis as well as the 6 months after their suicidal crisis. As seen in the figure, there were no significant pre–post differences in medical utili-zation for the CAMS patients. In contrast, there was a significant pre–post increase in medical utilization for the TAU patients. Moreover, the TAU patients had significantly more health care contacts than CAMS patients after seeking mental health care in our between-group analyses.

To further illustrate, the TAU group had 25 emergency room (ER) visits in the 6 months that followed their index mental health care while the CAMS group had 5 ER visits. These data suggest that CAMS care may also have significant implica-tions for risk and costs related to non-mental health medical utilization. But as noted in our article (Jobes et al., 2005), these data must be viewed with some cau-tion because direct causal attributions simply cannot be made from correlational data. Having said that, however, a series of *post hoc* reanalyses of the data examin-ing alternative "third variable" explanations for our findings (e.g., a clinician or site effect) revealed no overall differences in the major findings of the study. The

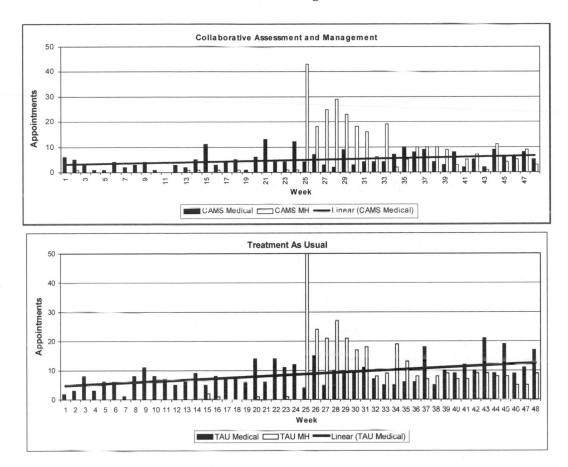

FIGURE 2.7. Interrupted time-series analysis.

data from this preliminary work are quite exciting, but the meaning and ultimate implications are markedly limited by the retrospective nature of this medical record (archival) study. Nevertheless, beyond inferential statistics and issues of research methodology and internal validity, the fact that CAMS *worked* for clinicians in real-world clinics facing considerable real-world demands is the important take-home point.

During a follow-up training workshop that I conducted for Air Force personnel in Colorado Springs, I had the pleasure of meeting the clinicians who worked in the clinics where the CAMS study was done. While I was pleased about their uniformly positive feedback about using CAMS, I was most taken by their clear sense of excitement and empowerment. I could see that CAMS had given them an approach that they believed could actually make a life-saving difference in the lives of their patients. I recognized this feeling of empowerment as I remembered discovering this feeling, when CAMS was first developed. This sense of clinical empowerment in the face of suicidal risk is fundamental to what makes the

CAMS work—for both the clinicians and ultimately for the suicidal patient as well.

SUMMARY AND CONCLUSIONS

As noted earlier in this chapter, among suicide risk assessment tools, the SSF is markedly different. Its initial development and evolution were shaped by pragmatically driven clinical needs. Clinical research has further shaped different portions of the SSF as we continue to craft the tool. A critical event occurred when the idea of administering the SSF collaboratively occurred as this transition marked the birth of the CAMS approach, which now encompasses the assessment of suicide as well as the development of the suicide-specific treatment plan. In addition, further SSF forms provide important vehicles for tracking the ongoing risk, changes in the treatment plan, and clinical outcomes. I have taken pains to walk the reader through each section of the SSF as the tool is so central to the CAMS approach. This chapter concluded with a discussion of the early development of the CAMS approach and a brief review of some recent research in support of CAMS.

Interest in CAMS is growing for a variety of reasons. For example, CAMS is practical, is clinically accessible, does not dictate the clinician's treatment, and does not usurp the clinician's judgment. It is my hope that clinicians reading this book will find the approach to be a viable and flexible short-term way of sensibly and effectively addressing this significant clinical issue. As a practicing clinician I know that CAMS works—I have personally used it in dozens of cases with great success. As an empirical researcher, I am excited by our SSF data and recent CAMS results. There are now a number of peer-reviewed papers that have been published providing substantial empirical support for this line of work (Drozd et al., 2000; Eddins & Jobes, 1994; Jobes, 1995a, 2000, 2003; Jobes & Berman, 1993; Jobes et al., 1997, 2004, 2005; Jobes & Drozd, 2004; Jobes & Mann, 1999, 2000). Clearly, the challenges of working with suicidal patients in contemporary care are considerable—both clinician needs and patient needs are great. The growing interest in CAMS reflects an evolving recognition that this particular approach addresses many of the clinical challenges inherent in working with suicidal patients. In addition, CAMS also responds well to a wide range of clinician *and* patient needs. This book thus represents a fundamental effort to make this new approach available to help empower clinicians to give their suicidal patients the live-saving help they so desperately need.

CHAPTER 3

The Early Identification of Suicide Risk

Survey research has consistently demonstrated that across mental health disciplines, the number-one greatest fear that clinicians harbor is the prospect of losing a patient to suicide (Pope & Tabachnick, 1993). Given the anxiety that these cases evoke—and the seriousness of the issue—it makes sense for clinicians to be on their toes to quickly identify any suicidal risk so that appropriate treatment can be brought to bear. Yet the limited data on what clinicians actually do suggest that mental health practitioners do not tend to respond in either a prompt or a thorough manner with suicidal patients (Coombs et al., 1992). Such failures to quickly and thoroughly respond to suicidality put the patient's life in peril and in turn significantly make a mental professional vulnerable to malpractice liability should a tragedy ensue.

With an eye to these considerations, I made the early clinical identification of any potential suicide risk a central emphasis within the CAMS approach. Accordingly, this chapter discusses the topic of early identification of suicide risk on both a conceptual level and a concrete clinical procedural level. I devote an entire chapter to this subject because widely accepted theory and data show that many clinicians have strong—often aversive—feelings toward suicidal patients that may naturally interfere with effective clinical care and their willingness to address the topic (Jobes & Maltsberger, 1995). Thus, to fully contextualize the larger discussion of this chapter, it is important to appreciate what we know about attitudes and approaches that clinicians have toward these particular patients.

COMMON CLINICIAN ATTITUDES
AND APPROACHES TO SUICIDALITY

One of the best known papers in the field of suicidology is a seminal paper written by two psychoanalysts: John Maltsberger and Daniel Buie. Their 1974 *Archives of General Psychiatry* classic paper titled "The Suicidal Patient and Countertransference Hate" starkly laid out the case that there is a unique set of negative feelings that clinicians harbor toward suicidal patients. It is important to note the word "hate" in the paper's title. "Hate"—certainly stronger than "dislike" or "unpleasant feelings toward"—was used on purpose to emphasize the intensity of feelings that clinicians often have toward their suicidal patients. Moreover, these authors describe a matrix of countertransferential reactions and behaviors that express deep feelings of *malice* and *aversion* in the clinician. In this important early paper, Maltsberger and Buie spoke plainly and directly to the strong negative feelings that clinicians often have that may directly undermine their ability to treat suicidal patients effectively.

For many years this theoretical paper has been quoted and referenced as virtual clinical fact—the paper is well written and intuitively compelling, but the ideas and the theory itself had never been empirically validated. Accordingly, three of my PhD students endeavored to empirically test the central components of Maltsberger and Buie's theoretical approach in their doctoral dissertations. Frankly, we found that empirically investigating the theoretical constructs of this psychoanalytic approach was quite challenging. The more we tried to quantify and empirically investigate the constructs of the theory, the more the constructs tended to lose the richness of their clinical meaning. We nevertheless persevered in our attempts to study countertransference reactions that were unique to suicidal patients through both analogue and survey studies (Crumlish, 1996; Jacoby, 2003). However, neither of these studies was able to robustly demonstrate that clinicians do in fact feel differently toward suicidal patients in comparison to other (nonsuicidal) difficult patients.

However, one unpublished dissertation study did find differences in how clinicians actually talked about suicidal patients (Judd, Jobes, Arnkoff, & Fenton, 1999). In this study we had undergraduate blind raters evaluate 80 verbatim transcripts of clinicians presenting cases of patients within a weekly case conference at the Chestnut Lodge Hospital in Maryland. We had our blind undergraduate coders evaluating the initial verbatim case presentation by the clinician (i.e., when they first talked about their patient within this professional format). Critically, half the sample ($n = 40$) was suicidal and eventually died by suicide, whereas the other half of the sample ($n = 40$)—matched for gender, diagnosis, and age—were neither suicidal nor died by suicide. While the effects were not overwhelming, we did find some statistically significant differences in the ways that clinicians talked negatively about their suicidal patients within the case conference setting, providing at least some empirical support for the Maltsberger and Buie's theory.

Beyond theory and research, many clinicians in practice forthrightly acknowledge having strong feelings about working with a range of difficult patients, particularly those who are suicidal. Through my extensive workshop training experiences, I am routinely struck by the intensity of feelings that clinicians have about these patients. As a reminder from Chapter 1, the clinical concerns with suicidal patients are fairly obvious—for example, suicidal states are difficult to assess and treat; our hands are tied by managed care; and plaintiff's attorneys are always lurking, waiting to litigate for wrongful death when we fail to prevent suicides. All these types of considerations contribute to an understandable wariness that many clinicians harbor toward these patients. But because suicidal presentations are common and the implications are so profound, we must find alternative ways of handling these adverse reactions to these patients so we can provide effective interventions.

Another challenge we face in contemporary care is that many of us were originally trained to immediately hospitalize any patient who mentions the topic of suicide (as noted in Chapter 1). With managed care restricting admissions and lengths of hospital stays, we must find ways to form a deeper *outpatient* engagement and a meaningful interpersonal connection with the suicidal patient. Israel Orbach (2001) has persuasively argued that if we truly hope to succeed with any suicidal patient, we must first find a way to be "empathic of the suicidal wish." By being empathic of suicidal desires, we open the door to connecting and to collaborating *without* necessarily endorsing suicide as a means of coping with pain and suffering. As I have discussed elsewhere (Jobes & Maltsberger, 1995), the key is to be engaged as a *therapist participant* who leads with empathic fortitude when working with suicidal patients—decidedly *not* the empathic dread of the "therapist voyeur."

The need to shift our attitudes and approach to suicidal patients (and the related consideration of hospitalization) cannot be overemphasized. As noted in Chapter 1, I have gone through a shift in attitude and approach as my own career has evolved, particularly because most of my early training occurred within psychiatric inpatient settings. However, as my professional clinical training progressed as an outpatient psychotherapist, I became increasingly aware of some strong fears and anxieties—my own countertransferential feelings toward my suicidal patients. As I came to understand these complex feelings, they were mostly rooted in my anxieties of not being able to ultimately control the potentially life-threatening behaviors of the patient and the implications of a patient actually ending his or her life under my care. Of course, these fears and anxieties are not at all unique to me. Again from my workshop perspective, clinicians routinely describe similar fears and related concerns. Bottom line, like many of my colleagues, I had a deep dread that even if I performed an excellent clinical assessment of suicide risk and provided outstanding treatment, the suicidal patient may *still* die by suicide.

But my perspective evolved as I learned more about suicidal states from my patients, and more about effective clinical assessments and possibilities for treatment. Through my empirical research that led to increasing my understanding of the suicidal mind, I was better able to understand what competent clinical work can actually do with a suicidal person. With knowledge came confidence, as I found that the fears and anxieties I had originally felt began to change. What I came to realize was that with knowledge and the proper clinical tools we can significantly improve the odds, rendering the prospect of completed suicide as highly unlikely. Suicidal patients are not typically hopeless cases that deserve to be shunned and avoided; rather, clinical experience and empirical findings have shown me that most suicidal people have lost track of making their lives viable and respond well to thoughtful clinical care. This gradual shift in perception and attitude led me from a place of fear and worry to a place of relative confidence and clinical competence.

Variations of this kind of shift in attitude and approach and this kind of thinking toward suicidal patients have been discussed elsewhere by other like-minded clinical suicidologists—refer to the work of colleagues such as Tom Ellis (2004), Shawn Shea (1999), Konrad Michel (e.g., Michel, Valach, & Waeber, 1994), Antoon Leenaars (2004), and the previously mentioned Israel Orbach (2001) and John Maltsberger (1994). In addition, a subgroup of clinician-researchers sponsors a biannual series of professional conferences that are held in Aeschi, Switzerland, to further develop alternative ways of working empathically with suicidal patients. As a charter member of the "Aeschi Group," I am pleased to say that the work of this like-minded group of colleagues has made a meaningful mark on the field through its website (www.aeschiconference.unibe.ch/), publications (e.g., Michel et al., 2002), and the biannual Aeschi conferences. The enthusiastic feedback we receive from conference participants of the Aeschi conferences makes clear that there is a deep commitment among clinicians to find new and better ways of clinically working with suicidal patients.

My own work in this area of attitudes and approaches to suicidality has been central to the development of CAMS (refer to Jobes, 1995a, 2000, and Jobes & Drozd, 2004). As suggested early on, the CAMS approach conceptualizes the assessment and treatment of suicidal patients in a fundamentally different way than current conventional approaches. CAMS is inherently designed to help shift clinicians' attitudes and approaches by changing our conceptualization of suicide as a clinical problem and thereby changing how we assess and treat this problem.

As shown in Figure 3.1, suicidality has been traditionally viewed as a *symptom* of some central psychiatric illness such as major depression. As depicted in Figure 3.1, clinical treatment within this model of care has typically focused on targeting the major psychiatric illness with the assumption that treating the illness will reduce the symptom of suicidal ideation and behaviors. In a contemporary sense this has often come to mean simply prescribing medication for the major illness with the expectation that successful treatment of the illness will include the reduction of suicidality. However, this assumption may not necessarily hold if we consider the extant literature on the treatment of suicidality as well as data pertaining to patients' poor compliance related to taking their prescribed medication (refer to discussions by Jobes & Drozd, 2004; Linehan, 1998; Rudd et al., 1999). Moreover, there is virtually no empirical support that medication alone has a meaningful impact on suicidal *behaviors* (Linehan, 2005).

More to the point, what I find to be particularly problematic about a reductionistic ("Kraepelinian") approach to suicide risk is the relational dynamic created between clinician and patient. Within this approach, the clinician is the active expert in a figurative "one-up" position, whereas the patient is a passive recipient of, and responder to, the clinician's largely diagnostically oriented questions. The clinician having made the diagnosis, then proceeds to treat the psychiatric illness—the patient is again placed in a passive recipient position.

But as illustrated in Figure 3.2, the CAMS approach takes a completely different approach to the situation. Within the CAMS conceptual framework and relational dynamic, *suicidality* is understood as the central clinical problem and

TRADITIONAL DIRECTIVE MODEL

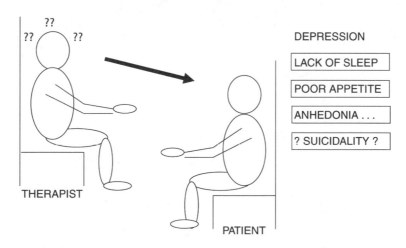

FIGURE 3.1. The Kraepelinian reductionistic approach to suicide. From Jobes (2000). Copyright 2000 by The Guilford Press. Adapted by permission.

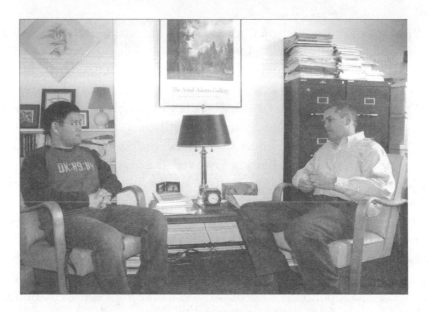

Traditional clinician as expert

focus. Moreover, while not ignoring legitimate concerns about psychiatric ill-ness, CAMS emphasizes the importance of understanding broader underlying issues (e.g., psychological suffering or self-hatred) that are *suicide-specific*. In this sense, directly assessing, targeting, and treating these underlying suicide-specific components—which lie at the heart of the patient's suicidality—may help the clinician and patient to systematically dismantle the meaning and value of suicide in the patient's struggle, thus rendering suicide obsolete as a means of coping

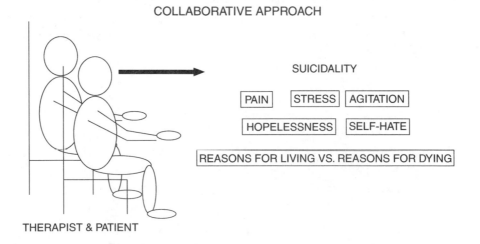

FIGURE 3.2. The CAMS conceptualization of suicidality. From Jobes (2000). Copyright 2000 by The Guilford Press. Reprinted by permission.

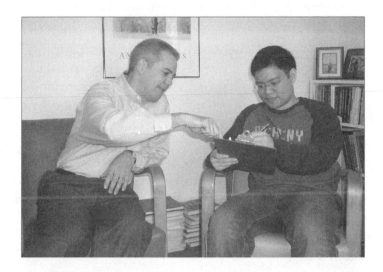

**The CAMS approach—the patient's perspective on suicidality
is the assessment gold standard.**

with pain and suffering (Jobes, 2000). In other words, CAMS emphasizes an assessment deconstruction of the suicidal risk that provides guidance and direction for treatment reconstruction of new and alternative ways of coping with pain.

Most critically, however, the CAMS relational dynamic is one of collaboration, where the patient—who is the expert of his or her own experience—is engaged as an active collaborator in clinical care. By literally taking a seat next to the patient to both clinically assess and treatment plan with the patient, the clinician communicates a completely different message to the patient: "The answers to your struggle lie within you—together we will find those answers and we will work as treatment partners to figure out how to make your life viable and thereby find better alternatives to coping than suicide."

By taking this clinical attitude and approach, the issue of suicidality is *objectified*—it is an issue that is mutually targeted with the patient. In this sense rather than approaching the suicidal patient with a sense of wariness—as a potential threat or adversary—CAMS facilitates a therapeutic alliance in relation to the issue of potential suicidal risk. Rather than being in a power struggle over whether the patient can take his or her life, CAMS averts the struggle with an alternative proposition: "Let us see if together we can find a viable alternative to suicide to better deal with your pain and suffering." In this manner, by avoiding the power struggle over whether the patient can take his or her life, the CAMS clinician seeks to form a meaningful relationship that ultimately can inspire the most essential ingredient for clinical success—*the patient's motivation to fight for life.*

Thus, the opening segment of this chapter has been written to both introduce and orient the reader to a fundamentally different clinical approach and attitude toward the suicidal patient that is central to the CAMS approach. I understand that simply reading about changing one's clinical approach and attitude is not sufficient to actually shift one's approach. To truly shift one's perceptions and approach initially requires awareness, but ultimately this shift requires a risk: to approach the issue (and patient) differently in order to garner the experience of success and the priceless dividend of clinical confidence that comes with success. One of the most satisfying experiences of developing CAMS and sharing the approach with other clinicians is the excited feedback I hear when a clinician has tried the approach and experienced the collaborative dynamic of CAMS (which by design erases the power struggles that so many of us have previously experienced with suicidal patients).

PRACTICAL CLINICAL IMPLICATIONS

Having explored clinician attitudes and approaches to suicidal patients, it is important to shift our attention to how we go about identifying suicidal risk early in the clinical encounter. For CAMS to succeed, it is crucial that any potential suicidal risk is identified as early as possible, *not* in the last 5 minutes of the clinical hour. To do this clinicians can use either a symptom-based screening tool or an interview. In the Air Force outpatient clinics where we did our previously described CAMS research, clinicians were encouraged to address the topic of suicide in the first 5 minutes of meeting with a potentially suicidal patient. This was relatively easy to achieve because in these clinics a symptom-based screening tool was routinely completed prior to each meeting with the clinician. In this manner, potential suicidal risk was captured by an assessment measure even before the patient crossed the threshold of the clinician's office. It is my strong recommendation that clinicians should consider the routine use of a multi-item symptom-based assessment screening tool to assess suicidal risk at the earliest possible juncture.

I recognize that some clinicians have an aversion to purchasing and using a symptom-based assessment tool. Importantly, choosing not to use such a measure does not preclude using CAMS with suicidal patients. Although I think it is the preferable way to go, I can attest that in the various clinics in which we have done our research—the Air Force, university counseling centers, and some inpatient settings—the initial implementation of using these tools *usually* is wrought with some measure of start-up ambivalence or discomfort. But after such measures become a part of a clinical culture, the routine use of these assessment tools can be successfully integrated into practice life.

In the Air Force clinics in which we conducted our CAMS research, the Outcome-Questionnaire—45 (OQ-45) was administered at every clinical contact, the clinicians developed a facile ability to quickly evaluate the presession OQ in the hallway on their way to greeting the patient. At Johns Hopkins University Counseling Center, the routine use of the Behavioral Health Measure (BHM) in advance of every session is deeply ingrained into the culture of the agency. I know in both these settings, from a purely administrative perspective, that routine collection of clinical data through such tools makes it much easier when JCHAO comes calling or when a counseling center director has to write an annual report. Of course, the empirical research implications are profound and my research team has been the grateful beneficiary of symptom-based assessments when they are routinely used (Jobes et al., 1997, 2005; Kahn-Greene et al., 2006). Bottom line, in reference to our central concern about working with suicidal patients, routine use of such tools gives the clinician a heads up for initiating the identification of suicidal risk early on, which is crucial to CAMS success both philosophically and on a concrete procedural level.

The Use of Symptom-Based Screening Tools

Within medical health care it is routine for a doctor or nurse to check a patient's vital signs during a routine checkup—blood pressure, pulse, temperature, and respiration. In fact, we would think it odd if our vitals were not checked in the course of a routine physical checkup. Yet, within mental health care it is rare for us to routinely check some comparable version of "vital signs" that are relevant to psychological health. However, there are considerable advantages to routinely using a symptom-based assessment tool, not only in any initial assessment but also at every clinical contact over the course of care. I know that there are some discipline-specific differences in regard to using assessment tools. For example, unlike psychologists, social workers, counselors, nurses, and psychiatrists are not typically trained in psychological testing, test construction, or the use of various assessment tools. Yet, the symptom-based measures I am describing do not require specialized training to use—they tend to have obvious face validity. With exposure and use I have seen clinicians become very comfortable with such assessment tools even when it is not a part of their professional training. Moreover, it is important to note that while the use of these tools provides valuable clinical information, these measures also provide hard copies of additional medical record documentation that can potentially decrease the clinician's liability.

The following is a brief review of a few instruments we have used in our research over the last 15 years. Each tool has strengths and limitations depending on the circumstances of their use. I describe our experiences with each and readers may determine for themselves what tool might be best for their practice. However, one clear virtue of each of the assessment measures is that they all have a suicide-specific question embedded among other symptom-based questions. When these measures are administered in advance of the session, the clinician can be readily alerted to the suicide risk potential thus creating the opportunity to address the issue of suicide early in the session.

Symptom Checklist–90

The measure first used in our SSF-based research at the Catholic University Counseling Center (Jobes et al., 1997) was the Symptom Checklist–90 (SCL-90). The original SCL-90 was a public domain assessment tool that was first developed by Derogatis and colleagues (Derogatis, Lipman, Rickels, Vhlenhuth, & Covi, 1974; Derogatis, Rickels, & Rock, 1976). The original scale provided a Global Severity Index of general symptom distress and various clinical subscales. Although the 90-item format was long and some patients complained about the overall length of the assessment, it was valuable tool for our pre–post treatment studies. Since the time of our initial research, Derogotis has improved the assessment tool by significantly decreasing the number of items to 53 and improving the structure and psychometrics of the clinical subscales (Derogotis & Savitz, 1999). The measure is now called the Brief Symptom Inventory (BSI). Research colleagues in Switzerland who are using a German translation of the BSI in the course of their CAMS-related work on an inpatient psychiatric unit report great clinical success using the measure; the potential research value of the assessment is clear according to our data analyses thus far. Critically, for our purposes, both the SCL-90/BSI have suicide-specific assessment questions that can be used from a presession administration to trigger CAMS with a suicidal patient.

Behavioral Health Measure

At the Johns Hopkins University Counseling Center we have used the Behavioral Health Questionnaire (BHQ) now called the Behavioral Health Measure (BHM) with great clinical and research success. The BHM was developed by Kopta and Lowry (2002) and is a 20-item self-report measure of general symptom distress. The BHM has been shown to have good to excellent construct validity, concurrent validity and test–retest reliability (ranging from .71 to.83; Kopta & Lowry, 2002). A clear merit of the BHM is that it is mercifully short and can be easily administered at every clinical contact. With multiple data points for any given course of treatment, the clinician can closely track the course of care both in terms of process and outcomes. From a research perspective, the routine and repeated use of the BHM at Johns Hopkins has enabled us to perform much more sophisticated linear analyses (e.g., hierarchical linear analyses—HLM) to understand treatment process and outcomes (Kahn-Greene et al., 2006). Like the SCL-90 and BSI, the BHM has a specific question about suicidal thoughts that we use as a trigger for CAMS in this counseling center setting. It is important to note that there are limits to using a shorter assessment tool such as the BHM. For example, the BHM does not capture as comprehensively more severe psychopathology. Although this is not particularly problematic in a higher-functioning university population, it may not be as quite well suited in other clinical settings where there is a broader range of psychopathology.

Outcome-Questionnaire–45.2

Another symptom based tool that is short enough to be administered at every clinical contact is the OQ-45 developed by Lambert, Hansen, and colleagues (1996). The OQ-45.2 is a 45-item self-report measure that again provides an over-all measure of symptom distress as well as three subscales that address (1) subjective discomfort, (2) interpersonal relationships, and (3) social role functioning. The OQ has good internal consistency ($r = .93$; Lambert, Hansen, et al., 1996) and test–retest reliability—at 3 weeks, the test–retest value is $r = .84$ (Lambert, Burlingame, et al., 1996). Lambert and colleagues further report that the OQ has good concurrent validity and sensitivity to treatment change in the course of care. Patients become quite familiar with the measure, especially with repeated administrations, and the OQ can be completed in only 5 minutes or less. In addition, there is also an online version of the OQ, which provides a useful alternative way of administrating the measure. I like the OQ for its range to handle the spectrum of psychopathology. The OQ item 8, "I have thoughts of ending my life," has been used with considerable success as a trigger item for CAMS and as a proxy index for suicidal ideation in our Air Force research (Jobes et al., 2005).

Interview-Based Identification of Risk

Having made the case for routine use of symptom-based assessment tools, I know that some clinicians may still opt not to use such measures in clinical practice for a variety of reasons. Clinicians who hold this view can of course discern potential current suicidal ideation through clinical interview. My only admonition, however, is to query about the possibility of suicidal ideation early in the interview, ideally within the first 5 to 10 minutes of the session. Without the waiting room "tipoff" of a symptom-based assessment tool, the clinician needs to be even more determined to ask the patient questions about current ideation before too much time lapses in the session.

PREPARATIONS FOR USING CAMS

To successfully launch the CAMS approach, the clinician needs to be able to move seamlessly from the early identification of current suicidal thoughts (via screening or interview-based query) to the introduction of a more thorough CAMS-based assessment of suicidal risk using the SSF. This means the clinician must literally have a hard copy, or an electronic version, of the SSF readily available before the session begins. In addition, the side-by-side seating that is used during CAMS assessment and treatment planning with the patient must be anticipated. This consideration is both philosophically and symbolically important in that literally getting up out of one's seat to sit adjacently to the patient is a significant thing to do. In CAMS, the patient is not talked down to; rather, he or she is collaboratively engaged as a therapeutic partner.

The side-by-side seating approach of the CAMS approach was in part inspired by the administration of the Rorschach Inkblot Test. Early in my career, I regularly administered the Rorschach and ended up teaching the test as part of an assessment course in our clinical psychology PhD program. Administering the Rorschach requires side-by-side seating as the examiner and examinee work together to complete the assessment. Over the years I have often been struck by the dynamic of this assessment administration. Central to administering the Rorschach is an emphasis on seeing the patient's percepts *through the eyes of the patient*.

In the course of using CAMS, I believe that the act of moving from the clinician's chair to an adjacent seat as a true collaborator with the patient has a significant impact on the clinical relationship. This was particularly true in the Air Force, where typically the move was further dramatized by the fact the doctor was an officer and the patient was usually an enlisted member of the service. In psychotherapy these kinesthetics are not trivial—consider, for example, how significant it is to psychoanalysis to have the patient (referred to as the analysand) lie on a couch with the analyst sitting behind. Obviously, the physical office space and chair arrangement must therefore be able to facilitate some version of the collaborative side-by-side seating that is used in CAMS. But taking a seat next to the patient is never to be done lightly. It must be done only with the patient's permission and with sensitivity to personal space, perceived status, and gender dynamics.

SUMMARY AND CONCLUSIONS

CAMS is fundamentally designed to change our orientation to the issue of suicide and finding ways of aligning with a patient in the midst of a life and death struggle. The collaborative emphasis in CAMS underscores the importance of seeing the world through the patient's eyes and forming a more viable therapeutic alliance. On a practical level, early identification of suicidal risk within CAMS may involve the use of symptom-based screening tools. Alternatively, the clinician can make verbal queries that can launch the assessment and treatment planning phase of CAMS in the index session. Most important, however, there is a relational dynamic that is struck when the clinician seeks permission to take a seat next to the patient to collaboratively complete the SSF with the patient. This symbolic and therapeutic move requires preparation on the clinician's part and a seating arrangement that allows for it.

CHAPTER 4

CAMS Risk Assessment

The Collaborative Use of the SSF

In many respects Chapter 4 is one of the most important chapters in this book. As previously noted, central to the CAMS approach to suicidality is the idea that a well-performed clinical assessment is invariably therapeutic, alliance forming, and motivation enhancing. In this chapter, I discuss both conceptual aspects and concrete procedural steps pertaining to the CAMS approach to suicide risk assessment. Because *how* this assessment is performed is so important, I provide scripted examples of what the CAMS clinician might say at each point in the assessment process. To be clear, although I am not suggesting that the assessor follow these scripts verbatim, these examples of what to say should nevertheless prove to be helpful in terms of underscoring certain philosophical and procedural aspects of the CAMS approach.

STEP-BY-STEP INSTRUCTIONS FOR CAMS RISK ASSESSMENT

The previous chapter discussed at length the importance of identifying suicidal ideation early in the clinical hour, particularly in the case of engaging a new patient. Clinical experience and our research have shown that the initial CAMS assessment and treatment planning phase in the index session takes at the very minimum at least 30–40 minutes, but a full 50 minutes is more usually required. As previously noted, because of this purely time-based consideration, the early identification of suicidal risk is very important and optimally triggered by a completion of a presession symptom-based screening tool. In this regard, to successfully use CAMS, clinicians must focus on the topic of suicide risk within the first *5–10 minutes* of the session, whether they use a symptom screening tool or not.

Many clinicians react negatively to the idea of "forcing" a focus on suicidal risk so early in a clinical contact, particularly if it is a first encounter with a new patient. Skeptical clinicians may say such a direct approach about such a sensitive issue could be offputting and a distraction to what the patient is prepared to talk about. Yet if the potential for suicidal risk is not clinically significant or relevant, the clinician and patient can move on to whatever else the patient wants to talk about. In other words, we have everything to gain and nothing to lose—the clinician undoubtedly makes things much more difficult by potentially putting off a direct focus on suicide.

CAMS by design is fundamentally devised to be alliance enhancing by emphasizing a collaborative clinical effort between the clinician and patient. CAMS directly facilitates a structured assessment opportunity to delve deeply into the patient's psychological pain and suffering, which is the front-end emphasis of CAMS. While significant and current suicidal ideation triggers the CAMS administration of the SSF, the initial focus of the assessment is much more on psychological pain and suffering than on suicide. Actually, specific questions about suicide come later in the process, toward the end of the SSF assessment. Whereas the topic of suicide can indeed be a bit sensitive for some patients, the rapid transition into a deep and meaningful discussion of pain and suffering is usually very well received and actually quite comforting. But *how* the clinician introduces the SSF is crucial for success.

Addressing the Topic of Suicide Risk

As previously discussed, before meeting with a patient for the first time, the clinician will know about the potential of current suicidal ideation in the patient by virtue of the completed symptom-based screening form that was completed in the waiting room. Accordingly, the clinician will have an SSF readily available and will start the session with a brief overview discussion about confidentiality and the HIPAA-compliant consent form that they have just signed in the waiting room. A typical question a clinician may ask to start the session could be, *"What brings you in to see me today?"* The patient will then characteristically present initial complaints, concerns, and symptom-related problems. Allowing the patient up to 5 minutes to describe what they are going through, the clinician may transition to the topic of suicide risk in the following manner:

> "It sounds like there is a lot going on for you right now and I am glad that you
> came in for help. It seems like you are overwhelmed and that you are in a

great deal of pain. It also appears that it is so difficult for you right now that you have actually had thoughts of suicide—based on the assessment form you completed in the waiting room. Because I understand such thoughts as a very serious indicator of how bad things are for you, I would like to conduct a deeper and more thorough assessment of your psychological pain and emotional suffering. To that end, I have an assessment tool here that I would like for us to complete together that I think we will find to be very helpful to us. Would it be okay if I move my chair next to you, so that we can work on this assessment together?"

I want to highlight a few key features of this passage. First, I always want to reassure the patient that it was a good idea to seek help—we should be hope vendors to our patients, affirming them in their decision to seek care. Second, I always make it clear that I empathically recognize the patient's sense of being utterly overwhelmed and that I understand that the patient has profound emotional suffering because he or she needs to hear that I understand the magnitude of the situation. Third, my reference to suicide is meant to be forthrightly interpreted as an emblematic proxy (an index) of how difficult and painful the situation has become—that suicide is understandable given the magnitude of their pain. Fourth, I purposely shift our clinical focus by emphasizing a need of a deeper assessment of the patient's *pain and suffering* that will be completed *together*, which will be helpful to us in our efforts to address the patient's pain and suffering. Fifth, I respectfully ask to take a seat adjacent to the patient to complete the SSF; I want the patient to know that I assume nothing; his or her comfort and willingness to proceed is a paramount concern of mine.

At this juncture, I would like to note that step-by-step instructions are difficult to relate to in the absence of clinical case material. I know well from my workshop training experiences that it is crucial to clinicians to hear about actual cases, to make theory, data, and the abstract come clinically alive. To address this need, I will use one of our published Air Force research cases to illustrate the initial completion of SSF Sections A and B (in this current assessment chapter) as well as Section C (in our next chapter on treatment). I have also included in Appendix E the entire "A–Z" SSF documentation for one of my first CAMS cases in order to more fully illustrate the complete SSF record within CAMS. It is my sense that these model cases will help make completion of the SSF and the process of CAMS much clearer and less abstract.

Filling Out Section A of the SSF

Once the clinician is seated next to the patient and the SSF is available on a tablet or clipboard, a brief overview of the form follows. For example, I typically say:

"This is an assessment tool called the Suicide Status Form. By completing each part of the form, we're going to get a better understanding of your emotional pain and suffering, which is currently making you feel suicidal. While we're going through this assessment, please feel free to ask me any questions. I'll be helping you complete the assessment and I will likely ask some questions along the way to help clarify some of your responses. The point of the first page of the SSF is for you to think about your suicidal struggle in a very focused way. That way, we can get a clearer sense of how you're feeling right now."

SSF Likert Ratings

The patient begins the SSF assessment by completing the six SSF Likert scales (i.e., Pain, Stress, Agitation, Hopelessness, Self-Hate, and Behavioral Risk). With each of the first five SSF constructs, the patient is further encouraged to write in his or her qualitative responses to each of the SSF Likert prompts. During the Section A phase of assessment, the clinician serves as consultant, coach, and collaborator—clarifying any questions the patient may have and assisting in the patient's efforts to complete the form. It is fine for the patient to leave some of the write-in responses blank (nonresponses can actually be useful data). The clinician should encourage the patient and help the patient to not get bogged down on any particular item. At the end of the Likert scale ratings, the clinician directs the patient to rank the order of the SSF constructs from 1 to 5 (most to least important).

To illustrate, let us consider a CAMS case seen in the course of our U.S. Air Force life skills outpatient mental health clinic research (refer to Jobes & Drozd, 2004). This case involved a 22-year-old active-duty married airman with complaints of depression secondary to multiple life stressors including marital, occupational, and financial problems. On his initial OQ-45 screening, the patient's rating for question 8, "I have thoughts of ending my life," was "frequently." I refer to this case throughout this chapter (and into the next) as a means of illustrating and clarifying the use of the SSF in CAMS. As we progress through the first two pages of the SSF using this particular case, I comment on various issues as they emerge from the SSF.

In this case example it is plain that the patient is in a great deal of pain over his work and marriage. In relation to Shneidman's Cubic Model of Suicide, we see ratings of "5" on Psychological Pain, "5" on Stress, and "3" on Agitation—a 5–5–3 rating. Although not as worrisome as a 5–5–5 rating (i.e., our operational definition of clear and imminent danger), we still see a very worrisome level of risk. Thankfully, his Agitation rating is somewhat lower, which in my mind is encouraging because agitation is such a lethal force; in other words the urgency here is not as high as his Pain and Stress, which gives us a preliminary sense that outpatient work might be possible with a well-crafted treatment plan and a solid Crisis Response Plan (which are further discussed in our next chapter). Upon completing the core SSF Likert ratings and qualitative responses, the patient rates the rank order of the core constructs. His number-one issue is Psychological Pain, which is followed by Hopelessness, Stress, Self-Hatred, and Agitation, respectively. I am again somewhat encouraged that Agitation is ranked 5.

Self versus Other Orientation to Suicide

The next two questions of Section A of the SSF shift the assessment focus from rating Likert scales to whether the patient's suicidal risk is oriented toward him- or herself or others (both or neither). As shown in the example case depicted in Figure 4.1, you can see that the patient is somewhat more self-oriented in his suicidal preoccupation, with no focus on others. This assessment is relevant to earlier theorizing in relation to *intrapsychic* versus *interpsychic* suicidal states (Jobes, 1995a). In the former case a patient is very internally focused in relation to psychological pain. In the latter case, interpsychic suicidal people's pain is much more relationally focused. It follows within this theory that intrapsychic suicidal patients are more at risk for completing suicide whereas interpsychic patients are more at risk for attempting suicide. Paradoxically, the theory and some of our data suggest that intrapsychic suicidal patients are probably less likely to seek treatment but more rapidly responsive to care if they do. Conversely, interpsychic suicidal patients are more likely to seek care but may be much more refractory to standard mental health treatments (Jobes, 1995a; Jobes et al., 2005—see also work by Fazaa & Page, 2005).

In specific reference to the Air Force case example, I would note that the patient is apparently not intent on making an interpersonal statement to anyone by his potential suicide; he is more preoccupied with his internal suffering. According to the theory, we would be concerned that his risk may be higher for completing versus attempting suicide, but the good news is that he may be a good candidate to quickly resolve his suicidality with intensive short-term care.

Reasons for Living versus Reasons for Dying

The focus of the SSF assessment next shifts to the RFL versus RFD assessment. This section is completed in any fashion that suits the patient. For example, some patients begin with RFD and only reluctantly, with the clinician's encouragement, shift their attention to RFL. To complete this section properly, the patient should fill in as many spaces as possible, but they are not required to fill every space.

SUICIDE STATUS FORM–III (SSF III) INITIAL SESSION

Patient: _____ Clinician: _____ Date: _____ Time: _____

Section A (*Patient*):

Rank | Rate and fill out each item according to how you feel <u>right now</u>.
Then rank items in order of importance 1 to 5 (1 = most important to 5 = least important).

Rank	
1	1) **RATE PSYCHOLOGICAL PAIN** (*hurt, anguish, or misery in your mind;* **not** *stress;* **not** *physical pain*): **Low Pain:** 1 2 3 4 ⑤ :High Pain What I find most painful is: *being stuck, trapped by myself at night in the box*
3	2) **RATE STRESS** (*your general feeling of being pressured or overwhelmed*): **Low Stress:** 1 2 3 4 ⑤ :High Stress What I find most stressful is: *everything, my wife bitching at me*
5	3) **RATE AGITATION** (*emotional urgency; feeling that you need to take action;* **not** *irritation;* **not** *annoyance*): **Low Agitation:** 1 2 ③ 4 5 :High Agitation I most need to take action when: *I'm by myself at night thinking—to stop thoughts*
2	4) **RATE HOPELESSNESS** (*your expectation that things will not get better no matter what you do*): **Low Hopelessness:** 1 2 3 4 ⑤ :High Hopelessness I am most hopeless about: *being alone, she's going to take off when I'm at work*
4	5) **RATE SELF-HATE** (*your general feeling of disliking yourself; having no self-esteem; having no self-respect*): **Low Self-Hate:** 1 2 3 ④ 5 :High Self-Hate What I hate most about myself is: *the way I act, I'm miserable all the time*
N/A	6) **RATE OVERALL RISK OF SUICIDE:** **Extremely Low Risk:** 1 2 3 ④ 5 :Extremely High Risk (will <u>not</u> kill self) (will kill self)

1) How much is being suicidal related to thoughts and feelings about <u>yourself</u>? **Not at all:** 1   2   3   ④   5 :completely
2) How much is being suicidal related to thoughts and feelings about <u>others</u>? **Not at all:** ①   2   3   4   5 :completely

Please list your reasons for wanting to live and your reasons for wanting to die. Then rank in order of importance 1 to 5.

Rank	REASONS FOR LIVING	Rank	REASONS FOR DYING
1	*wife*	*1*	*stop thinking*
3	*want kids some day*	*2*	*wife wouldn't have to deal with me*
4	*friends*		
2	*parents*		

I wish to live to the following extent: **Not at all:**   0   1   2   3   ④   5   6   7   8   :Very much
I wish to die to the following extent: **Not at all:**   0   1   2   3   4   ⑤   6   7   8   :Very much

The one thing that would help me no longer feel suicidal would be: *to keep my wife* _____

FIGURE 4.1. Example of completed SSF, page 1.

53

Following the listing of responses, the patient is asked to rank-order the items from most to least important (1 to 5 for each side of the assessment—RFL and RFD, respectively). As with all SSF qualitative assessments, it is not crucial for the patient to complete all five RFL/RFD spaces with responses.

In reference to the case, we see completely relationally oriented RFL pertaining to his wife, friends, parents, and the prospect of children some day. These are very encouraging RFLs because they tell us that we have some resources to work with in the interpersonal sphere. In other words, I am already thinking about the possibility of interventions involving his wife, friends, and parents—he has told us in his own words that they are people who make him want to live. The reference to having children is very encouraging as well as a quintessential plan/goal for the future. Our research shows that evidence of *any* expressed future thinking on any part of the SSF is always noteworthy and may function as a protective factor (Jobes, 2004b; Nademin et al., 2005).

Wish to Live versus Wish to Die

Upon completion of the RFL/RFD assessment, the patient is then encouraged to complete the 0–8 Likert ratings pertaining to wishes to live versus wishes to die. This assessment is based on Kovacs and Beck's (1977) "internal struggle hypothesis"—recent work by Brown, Steer, and colleagues (2005) has further demonstrated the utility of this assessment.

Referring back to the case example, we see the classic ambivalence of a very suicidal person. The ratings reflect a relatively high wish to live ("4" on a 9-point scale); however, the wish to die rating is a point higher ("5"), suggesting that the scale is tipped toward dying—but not egregiously.

SSF One-Thing Response

The final assessment under Section A of the SSF is the One-Thing response. Patients may respond to this query in any manner they prefer. For example, some patients will give more than one response. This is fine. The CAMS clinician should neither be too directive nor too restrictive in relation to how the patient completes any of the SSF qualitative assessments.

Again, referring back to the case example we see one of the virtues of the simple One-Thing assessment. There is in my mind no ambiguity as to what is a central preoccupation with this patient: his marriage. He is telling us in his own words—"to keep my wife"—the one thing that could make the difference around his ambivalence to live or die. At this juncture, is there any question as to what will be a central focus of his treatment? Obviously, trying to work on the marriage through some form of couple therapy is crucial.

Conclusion of Section A

Completion of Section A of the SSF typically takes from 15 to 25 minutes (in the case example it took 17 minutes to complete Section A). Completion of this first page of the SSF should not be rushed, but the patient and clinician should not get bogged down on any one portion of the assessment. There is an important balance between pushing the patient and getting too delayed thereby not moving through all the necessary materials in a timely and reasonable fashion. I cannot emphasize enough that the 15–25 minutes spent on completing Section A is critical for CAMS success. The process of engaging the patient—coaching, clarifying, and assisting—creates the crucial collaborative synergy that is the backbone of the CAMS approach to suicidality. Through this initial SSF assessment the CAMS therapeutic relationship dynamic is forged. It is in this crucial phase that an important and lasting impression is made on the patient: "I am genuinely interested in understanding your pain and suffering by seeing the world through your eyes."

Filling Out Section B of the SSF

After completing Section A, there is an important transition to Section B. The clinician remains seated next to the patient and takes the SSF back to complete Section B (the clinician's assessment section). As discussed in Chapter 3, this section contains a listing of key empirically based risk factors for suicide. To make this assessment transition and to further orient the patient to this phase of the SSF assessment process, the clinician may begin this phase by saying something like:

> "We have just finished an important part of our assessment and I feel like I have a much better understanding about the pain and suffering that has led you to feeling suicidal. There are now an additional set of questions that we must consider together. Taken together with the previous page, these assessment questions will help us come up with a workable plan for dealing with your suicidal pain and suffering."

It is important to move through the Section B questions with the patient in an even and steady fashion. Each question is posed to the patient in a matter of fact manner with no hint of judgment or any desired response in the clinician's voice. The patient looks on as the clinician completes Section B. Figure 4.2 shows the Section B continuation of the Air Force case example.

The following discussion addresses each of the empirically based assessment items in Section B so that the clinician is familiar with each question in order to make clarifications and to effectively gather this important and necessary assess-

SUICIDE STATUS FORM–III INITIAL SESSION (PAGE 2)

Section B (*Clinician*):

(Y) N Suicide Plan: When: *night shift*

Where: *gate*

How: *gunshot wound to head* (Y) N Access to means

How: ______ Y N Access to means

Y (N) Suicide Preparation Describe: ______

(Y) N Suicide Rehearsal Describe: *has put gun in mouth*

(Y) N History of Suicidality

- Ideation Describe: *recent ideation to shoot self*
  - Frequency *2–3* per day ______ per week ______ per month
  - Duration ______ seconds *30* minutes *2* hours
- Single Attempt Describe: *denies*
- Multiple Attempts Describe: *denies*

(Y) N Current Intent Describe: *wants to end pain/thoughts*

Y (N) Impulsivity Describe: ______

Y (N) Substance Abuse Describe: ______

Y (N) Significant Loss Describe: ______

Y (N) Interpersonal Isolation Describe: ______

(Y) N Relationship Problems Describe: *marital problems*

Y (N) Health Problems Describe: ______

Y (N) Physical Pain Describe: ______

Y (N) Legal Problems Describe: ______

Y (N) Shame Describe: ______

Section C (*Clinician*): **OUTPATIENT TREATMENT PLAN** (Refer to Sections A & B)

Problem #	Problem Description	Goals and Objectives Evidence for Attainment	Interventions (Type and Frequency)	Estimated # Sessions
1	*Self-Harm Potential*	*Outpatient Safety*	**Crisis Response Plan:** *Pt actively engaged in safety action planning*	*2x/week for 2 weeks*
2	*↓ depression*	*acquire/implement CBT strategies* *Rx consult*	*CBT + Rx*	*8*
3	*↑ couple's communication*	*speaker–listener technique*	*couple therapy*	*4*

YES ✓ NO ______ Patient understands and commits to outpatient treatment plan?

YES ______ NO ✓ Clear and imminent danger of suicide?

______ Patient Signature Date ______ Clinician Signature Date

FIGURE 4.2. Example of completed SSF, page 2.

ment information. I continue to refer to the Figure 4.2 responses to further illustrate key points in relation to our case example.

Suicide Plan

The plan for suicide is a critical initial consideration. We know from previous research and clinical experience that the clarity and concreteness of a suicidal plan are an important window into the seriousness of suicidal intent. In other words, someone with a vague, inexact, or nonspecific plan is much less serious about completing suicide. In marked contrast, a patient who is very specific and has a detailed plan, including a particular place, time, and date, is someone who is much more psychologically invested in suicide, reflecting a much more serious level of intent. To assess the level of suicide intent, the SSF prompts for additional information about the "when," "where," and "how" of the suicidal plan with an additional question about whether the patient has access to the means of the plan (i.e., does the patient have a stash of lethal pills or access to a firearm).

Referring back to our case example, this particular Section B SSF query led to a startling admission that the patient had been thinking about shooting himself in the head with his sidearm pistol, during his night-shift duty, while in his guard booth at the entry to the base. He acknowledged to the clinician that he had literally been sitting in the booth with the gun muzzle in his mouth praying to God for the strength to pull the trigger. This is an example of a very specific plan with a frighteningly clear when, where, and how revealing a significant level of suicidal intent. It should be further noted that the SSF suicide plan query can accommodate two separate suicidal plans, which is not unusual to see. While patients sometimes have additional plans, more than two plans is relatively rare.

Suicide Preparation

Many suicidal people engage in specific preparation behaviors prior to making an attempt or taking their life (refer to Rudd & Joiner, 1998). In general, preparation behaviors are often related to organizing the suicide attempt itself, such as the procurement of lethal means, doing research on the Internet to determine a lethal dose of drugs, or determining a suitable location where the possibility of interruption or intervention may be reduced. Other preparation behaviors may include putting one's affairs in order, writing a will, the writing of suicide notes, shooting a good-bye videotape, doing a favorite activity one final time, saying a final good-bye to friends and family, or giving away of prized possessions. All of these behaviors infer significantly increased risk, behaviorally "ramping up" to a suicidal act. In our case, there were apparently no particular preparation behaviors worthy of note.

Suicide Rehearsal

Separate from suicidal preparations are another related set of relevant behaviors referred to as rehearsal behaviors. These behaviors typically involve a literal acting out or playing through of the planned suicide attempt. For example, someone may hang a rope, find a beam in the garage, secure the rope at a certain length, position a short stool, and even step up on the stool and place the ligature around the neck without then stepping off the stool to make the attempt. Such rehearsal behavior is very serious—usually ending just short of the actual attempt behavior. Many completed suicides are known to have held loaded guns to their head, placing the barrel of the gun at different locations or perhaps having put the barrel into their mouth—as in our case example. Such behaviors are very important to identify as they represent the most dangerous of preparatory behaviors. Metaphorically, through their rehearsal behaviors, the patient walks up to the very precipice of death and teeters as he or she looks over the edge.

History of Suicidality

There is probably no better predictor of future suicidal behavior than the presence of past suicidal behavior. The work of Rudd and Joiner (1998; Joiner et al., 2005) has made clear that there are distinct differences between people who have only had suicidal thoughts versus those who have made a single attempt versus those who have made multiple attempts. The risk of prospective behavior increases significantly with any past attempt behaviors, particularly a multiple-attempt history. In this area, the clinician is assessing for primarily genuine attempts, not superficial sublethal acts of scratching or minor overdoses.

Referring back to the case example, the good news is that there is no apparent history of suicide attempts. The bad news is that there is a contemporary history of significant suicidal ideation—two to three times per day in durations lasting from 30 minutes to 2 hours! This is a very worrisome level of suicidal preoccupation, particularly because it occurs late at night in his guard booth, by himself, with a gun in his hand and sometimes in his mouth.

Current Intent

An obviously important assessment question centers on the patient's current intent in regard to suicidal thoughts. What is operative here is whether there is a clear intent to die. As we know, suicidal ideation is multifaceted. There are often interpersonal aspects to suicide—threats of suicide can profoundly mobilize the support of loved ones. Sometimes there is a need to just do something—

anything—rather than deal with seemingly unending pain and suffering. So there is always a basic question about what the psychological intent is when the patient considers suicide. In relation to the case example there is clear intent to end his pain and suffering (i.e., to put himself out of his own misery).

Impulsivity

Because completed suicides most often happen during highly impulsive states, often among people with a history of impulsivity, it is important to get a sense of the patient's historic and current impulsivity. Impulsivity can be characterized broadly in terms of a range of behaviors and actions that were not well thought through. The risk is further increased if such behaviors are inherently self-destructive. In other words, a history of fighting, conduct-based problems, and impulsive decision making that the patient later regrets is important to consider.

Fortunately, in our case example there is no apparent history of impulsivity. Combining this assessment with his apparent lack of agitation (from Section A assessment) is very promising from an imminent risk assessment standpoint. If I am the clinician, I am thinking that there may be some hope of working on an outpatient basis even though the risk is notable.

Substance Abuse

Another risk factor that is often implicated in suicidal behaviors is substance abuse. We know that substance abuse contributes significantly to increases in impulsive behaviors by lowering impulse control. Moreover, many people complete suicides in a state of intoxication. Among the major Axis I mental disorders, alcohol abuse is a very significant psychopathology diagnosis highly associated with suicide. No evidence of substance abuse is noted for the case example.

Significant Loss

For many years suicidologists have known that suicides are often precipitated by losses that seem to trigger the suicidal act. Such losses may be big or small; it can be one particularly significant loss or an accumulation of several lesser losses. Examples may include a marital divorce or a romantic breakup, a financial disaster, the death of a loved one or a pet—literally any tangible event that has meaning. Moreover, suicide-triggering losses can also be symbolic—for example, retirement from a meaningful career. Whatever the case, losses often contribute to the circumstances that precede the suicide; usually such losses are not singularly causal of a suicide. In relation to the case example, there are no apparent significant losses.

Interpersonal Isolation

Following the work of sociologists we know that social factors are meaningfully implicated in suicidal behaviors. Across the age spectrum we know that social relationships and social integration tend to protect a person against suicide. From a clinical intervention standpoint it is always important to endeavor to not let the highly suicidal person be alone. Although it is not specifically noted for the case, the fact that the patient sits by himself at night in the guard booth is very worrisome to me.

Relationship Problems

In a related but more specific sense, we know that most of the suicidal patients we have studied (Jobes et al., 2004) have relationships as their number-one suicide-related concern. These suicidogenic relationship problems may be romantically based or focused on friends or family (see also Joiner, 2005). We already know that within our case example, the marriage difficulties are a huge issue for the patient.

Health Problems

There are also data that suggest that general health-related issues, particularly if these issues are chronic, may be implicated in suicidal states (Maris et al., 2000). There are no apparent health problems in the case example.

Physical Pain

Chronic physical pain, in particular, is often linked to mental pain, which may in turn foster wishes for a suicidal escape. Unremitting chronic pain is a significant risk factor implicated in psychological autopsy research (Maris et al., 2000). There are apparently no physical pain issues in the case example.

Legal Problems

Legal problems can also contribute significantly to suicidal risk. Indeed, we know suicide attempts and completions among individuals in lockup or holding cells (oftentimes picked up for driving under the influence of alcohol) are a notable concern. There is often a window of considerable suicidal risk shortly after a person is first faced with a legal accusation (Oordt, Jobes, et al., 2005). There are no apparent legal problems for the patient depicted in the case example.

Shame

Finally, a related but unique risk factor is shame, which can play a key role in the need to escape seemingly unbearable discovery for past wrongs or experiences that cannot be borne in the eyes of others. For example, I know of cases of priests facing charges of child abuse who have attempted or completed suicide rather than face the misery of prolonged litigation that will be both professionally and personally humiliating. Conversely, being the victim of abuse can play a particularly pernicious role in suicidal and self-destructive behavior (Linehan, 1993). There are no apparent shame issues in the case example.

Conclusion of Section B

After completing Section B of the SSF, the clinician and patient are ready to transition to Section C of the SSF—the development of a suicide-specific treatment plan. In terms of wrapping up the index session SSF assessment, the clinician may say:

> "I appreciate your willingness to complete this assessment with me. I think we now both have a much better sense of what has been going on with you and why suicide has been on your mind. Knowing why you are suicidal is crucial to finding alternative ways of coping with your pain and suffering. Do you have any questions before we start working on your treatment plan?"

Case Example Risk Formulation. In relation to the case example of the suicidal airman, my summary assessment is that he clearly represents a considerable suicidal risk. Specifically, I would say that he is at a high risk for suicide given his degree of mental pain and suffering and his hopelessness, and particularly in relation to his recent history of rehearsal behaviors that include actually putting a loaded gun in his mouth while having serious and lengthy contemplations of ending his life. His marriage appears to be in significant trouble and his self-worth and future plans seemed closely linked to staying in this marriage. The patient hates his work, his love relationship is in crisis, and he hates the way he sees himself acting. All these considerations would obviously give me pause to seriously consider an immediate hospitalization.

However, within CAMS, a hospitalization even in the face of this kind of risk is not a given. As discussed further in our next chapter, whether this patient gets hospitalized really depends on the specificity and quality of the treatment plan and his commitment to his Crisis Response Plan and overall intent to fight for his life. I know that many clinicians would feel automatically compelled to try hospitalizing such a patient; the risk is considerable. However, a balanced assessment is necessary to see the full picture.

To this end, there is some SSF assessment-based data that are actually somewhat promising in this case, particularly in relation to certain issues that are *not* present. For example, if he had rated his agitation at a level of "5" and had a history of attempts or impulsivity, I would be thinking that a hospitalization would be warranted to ensure the airman's immediate safety. But there does appear to be some impulse control here. Although it is extremely worrisome that he contemplates suicide in episodes lasting up to 2 hours, that is still 2 hours of *not* acting in the presence of a lethal means. That means a lot. Moreover, the airman has some significant RFL—namely, his wife and other significant relationships who could be engaged (with his consent) in the short term as part of the Crisis Response Plan and possibly in his longer term ongoing treatment as well. In terms of the other empirically based risk variables in Section B, I am struck that there are no extensive risk factors in this case—this suicidal situation is contemporary, it is intense, but it can be largely understood as a first-time encounter of this kind of pain and suffering. Thus, I am very concerned about the risk in this case, but I have a tentative sense that using CAMS will enable me to see even a case as serious as this one on an outpatient basis.

SUMMARY AND CONCLUSIONS

As noted at the chapter's start, the completion of SSF Sections A and B in the index session is crucial to the success of CAMS. Everything about the CAMS approach to assessing suicide risk is meant to forge an alliance and engage the patient in care. The emphasis of Section A is meant to communicate that the patient is the expert of his or her own experience. It is the clinician's job to see the suicidal risk through the eyes of the patient. The patient's perceptions of the struggle are the assessment gold standard and the clinician's job is to appreciate and understand those perceptions. A case example from an active duty Air Force outpatient was used to illustrate and underscore the importance of seeing the suicidal struggle through the unique and idiosyncratic perceptions of the patient. As noted, Section A heavily emphasizes a focus on pain and suffering more than suicide. Having emphasized the patient's pain and suffering, Section B marks a transition to focusing very specifically on empirically based suicide risk factors. The backloading of the more suicide-specific focus of Section B makes this section secondary to the primary focus of the phenomenological emphasis of Section A. By performing the risk assessment this way, we underscore an empathic approach to working with the patient in an effort to sidestep the suicide-hospitalization/no-hospitalization power struggle. In so doing, we increase the likelihood of forming a collaborative alliance and inspiring motivation in the patient to fight for life as operationalized in the outpatient treatment plan.

CHAPTER 5

CAMS Treatment Planning

Coauthoring the Outpatient Treatment Plan

As we all know, there are literally hundreds of different types of psychotherapies represented in the clinical literature. When I first taught courses in our graduate program it was common to think in terms of the three major schools of theory: psychoanalytic, behavioral, and humanistic. Today, these major schools have further evolved and blended. For example, psychoanalytic theory has evolved into a variety of "psychodynamic" schools of thought, including ego psychology, drive theory, object relations, and self psychology to name but a few. Humanistic theories have perhaps waned a bit in popularity, but there are still enthusiastic practitioners of Rogerian and existential psychotherapies. Behavioral treatments, combined with cognitive approaches, have clearly been in ascension over the last decades and tend to have the best overall empirical support.

As an academic clinician I find myself firmly rooted in almost all of the above. I have never thought that there is one theoretical truth to which all patients fit. I tend to conceptualize psychodynamically but practice with more of a cognitive-behavioral bent, with a fair sprinkling of humanistic, interpersonal, and existential also in the mix. In other words, I am eclectic and integrative in my orientation. But I recognize that not all clinicians work this way, which could have been a potential problem when trying to develop a clinical approach like CAMS. Accordingly, my goal in developing CAMS was to create a methodology that could be widely used no matter what the clinician's theoretical encampment or treatment approach.

I ultimately concluded that to succeed in this goal, the treatment philosophy and clinical framework of CAMS must (1) cut across theoretical approaches, (2) be conducive to a range of techniques, and (3) ultimately accommodate virtually any larger theoretical orientation and approach to treatment. For example, clinicians who are psychodynamically inclined *and* those who are cognitive-behaviorally oriented should both be able to use CAMS with their suicidal patients without giving up their preferred world view of treatment. Thus, CAMS was specifically designed to handle all comers—there is no need to convert to an alternative theoretical camp or treatment approach to successfully use the flexible framework of CAMS with suicidal patients.

Nevertheless, using CAMS successfully with suicidal patients requires a certain appreciation and application of an important philosophical approach to *outpatient* treatment planning, which naturally flows from the preceding chapter on the CAMS risk assessment. In short, CAMS does have some front-end requirements for engaging, assessing, and treatment planning with suicidal patients, but thereafter the clinician can proceed to use virtually any theory or treatment that is appropriate. In this regard, I have often argued (e.g., Jobes & Drozd, 2004) that CAMS has been purposely designed to neither usurp clinical judgment nor dictate the theory or type of treatment that the clinician must use. To more fully walk the reader through the various considerations of the CAMS approach to treatment planning, the current chapter first considers some conceptual aspects of CAMS treatment planning before shifting the focus to step-by-step treatment planning procedures.

THE CAMS PHILOSOPHY
TO OUTPATIENT TREATMENT PLANNING

The CAMS approach to working with suicidality involves a certain kind of pragmatic clinical philosophy toward the whole professional undertaking of trying to help virtually any suicidal person. As discussed in Chapter 1, many of the ways we have learned to help suicidal patients clinically have proven to be unsatisfactory, particularly in more recent years. As I have noted, there is a contemporary need for an entirely new and effective approach to working with suicidal patients. Critically, I knew that such an approach would have to avoid the adversarial power struggles over hospitalization and the potentially stigmatizing effect that often comes with an inpatient hospitalization. I have never felt comfortable with the use of "no-suicide contracts," and like many of my colleagues I had considerable fears about malpractice litigation should I "fail" to save a suicidal patient. Plainly, suicidal patients leave many clinicians feeling clinically ill prepared and vulnerable.

CAMS is therefore designed to actually empower clinicians, by empowering patients. I was determined to develop an approach to help my suicidal patients fight for their life, before they felt inexorably compelled to take it. To achieve this goal, I knew I had to find an approach that, first, would help build the best possible clinical alliances and, second, would also inspire motivation in my patients. It follows that virtually every component of CAMS is directly or indirectly intended to maximize the potential for these two indispensable therapeutic ingredients to achieve clinical success in the face of suicidal risk.

What emerged in the early development of CAMS were two important insights: (1) among a person's options for dealing with unbearable pain and suffering is the blunt prospect of suicide, and (2) given this, it is crucial to clinically embrace the importance of developing transparent *time-specific* treatment plans to optimally help the suicidal person through the potential risk. Suggesting to a suicidal patient that suicide is not an option is both unempathic and simply not true. Each day approximately 85 Americans take their life. We may not like it, we may not morally approve, we may be clinically opposed (as I am), but the fact is that a determined person who means to die can achieve the goal of death by suicide. As discussed in Chapter 1, we clinicians no longer have the illusion that we can "lock up" a suicidal person until clinical stability is achieved. Managed health care simply prohibits lengthy hospital stays. Completed suicide is a frank clinical reality; it is a bottom line that demands our thoughtful attention and reflection.

When it comes to clinical care, you must ask yourself: "If suicide is obviously the best option for a person to cope with pain and suffering, *why is this person talking to me—a mental health professional?*" The answer invariably is that the person is talking to you because he or she has not yet decided that suicide is in fact the *best* way of coping with pain and suffering. Simply stated, such a person is undoubtedly ambivalent, and this ambivalence is the portal through which you can find life-saving clinical interventions.

While the suicidal patient is almost always ambivalent, the seduction of suicide is nevertheless extraordinarily powerful. In this regard, the clinician must skillfully manage the temporal aspects of negotiating the treatment plan with the suicidal patient. Time is the key. It is simply unreasonable for a highly suicidal person to give up suicide as an option for coping *indefinitely*. Alternatively, it is not unreasonable for a clinician to negotiate a discrete time period in which clinical treatment is given a fair chance, thus pushing the option of suicide onto the patient's psychological back burner. My foot-in-the-door argument to the patient is this: "Before you take your life to end your pain and suffering, let's try to give clinical treatment a reasonable chance to help you find other ways of coping— obviously, there are many options—like suicide—that you can reflect on later without my help."

The last portion of this statement may sound overly provocative. But in a clinical context with the proper tone and emphasis, such a statement is not only reasonable, it is also empathic and typically deescalates a potential power struggle.

Perhaps most notably, this statement and position does not eliminate from the already vulnerable patient his or her sense of power and control that the option of suicide psychologically promises. In my mind, one of the most powerful clinical interventions one can make when working with a suicidal person is to overtly negotiate with the patient the notion of putting off suicide to a later point in time. The issues are as follows: What is reasonable for the clinician to expect of a suicidal patient; in turn, what is reasonable, from the suicidal patient's perspective, in regard to further endurance of unbearable suicidal pain and suffering to explore the promise of treatment?

I assert to my suicidal patients that it is clinically reasonable and appropriate to negotiate suicide-specific outpatient treatment plans that are finite. In CAMS, patients are explicitly asked to commit to a mutually negotiated suicide-specific treatment plan for an exact period of time. Within CAMS there should *never* be clinical or moral coercion or an open-ended approach to treatment planning. As noted earlier, when I negotiate a suicide-specific treatment plan with a suicidal patient, I forthrightly acknowledge that the patient can obviously take his or her life *later* (when not otherwise engaged in treatment focused on saving that life). But I emphatically insist that while the patient is engaged in our suicide-specific time-limited treatment, the patient must be fully committed—as I will be—to that treatment. Typically this treatment thoughtfully explores, among other things, whether there are in fact viable alternatives to the finality of suicide.

I am always explicit with my patients that if they become a clear and imminent danger to self or others (as described in the HIPAA-compliant consent form that they read and signed before our first session), I will not hesitate to hospitalize them as per legal statutes that require clinicians to intervene in this manner. But anything short of this extreme medicolegal threshold leaves a great deal of wiggle room for the clinician and patient to thoughtfully maneuver as they collaboratively endeavor to negotiate a potentially life-saving treatment plan. I point out that the patient has everything to gain, and really nothing to lose, by giving treatment a chance. To succeed, it is imperative that patients believe that they are maintaining some sense of control by understanding that they can take their life later, *after* they have given treatment a fair and reasonable chance. Whenever I say things along these lines, I remain absolutely clear that I do not endorse suicide as a viable option and that I will never "sign off" on suicide as the desirable way to respond. Thus, patients are posed with a profound choice: Do they want to live a bit longer to see if treatment can help make their life livable without pain, or do they choose not to be in treatment and to continue to be subjected to unbearable suffering, with the obvious implications therein? It is a profound choice, but I think it must be plainly posed to the patient as such. I clearly think it is incumbent upon the clinician to skillfully pose to the suicidal patient a time-specific treatment option that compels an intentional decision to *choose to live*.

What follows is a metaphor I often use with my patients that captures part of what I am suggesting, which embodies a core philosophical notion about treatment within CAMS:

"I want you to consider taking a therapeutic road trip with me. On this trip you will be the driver and I will be the navigator. I have taken this trip many times before, I know the roads well and I have excellent maps. But the journey is never the same route for any two drivers, it is always unique to the driver and the way we decide to travel together—which roads to take, when to stop, and how fast or slow we decide to go. For this road trip to be successful, you must, like me, commit to the trip. I know that our desired therapeutic destination can be hard to find and frankly we may take some wrong turns along the way. But I nevertheless remain confident that we can get to where we want to go if we work together as a traveling team.

"Because I know you suffer deeply, I am only asking that you travel with me for a very specific period of time, a minimum of 4 weeks to a maximum of 3 months. At which point we can decide together whether we should continue our travels or perhaps part ways so that you can drive on your own or perhaps travel with a different navigator. In spite of your suffering, I still believe this is a reasonable request to ask of you given the promise of our desired destination and the seriousness of the alternative you are considering.

"If you agree to take this trip with me, for a period of time to which we can both commit, then it requires that we both seriously promise to pursue this journey. That means you must get completely in the car, with the door closed and locked, seat belt on, both hands on the wheel. This journey will fail if you insist on leaving your door ajar so that you may jump out of the car if the road gets bumpy. If that is something you need to do, then we need to find you another navigator or perhaps we should acknowledge that you are not yet ready to take this kind of trip with a person like me.

"As the navigator, I will stay right beside you with my expertise, maps, and experience to facilitate this trip for the period of time we are both committing to so that we may find the therapeutic destination that we both seek. I can assure you that the destination is a much better place than where you now reside, it will be a place where your pain and suffering is meaningfully decreased and your ability to cope with life is meaningfully improved. . . ."

I want to emphasize that to properly take this metaphorical journey, both parties must be fully seated in the car—no doors are open, no metaphorical feet are allowed to hang out. We are asking the patient to commit, and in turn, the patient can anticipate that we will commit as well, with both doors closed and seat belts securely fastened. We both commit to taking this therapeutic trip together in search of a prized location that the patient has clearly not been able to find up to this point traveling solo. For patients who are not up for taking this type of therapeutic trip under these travel conditions I indicate that there are basically three options: (1) an inpatient hospitalization if they are in imminent danger, (2) referral to another clinician who travels in a different manner with different traveling conditions, or (3) for the patient—*if not in imminent danger*—to continue driving on his or her own without my help (i.e., the obvious but often overlooked option of not being in mental health treatment).

As I have discussed elsewhere (Wise, Jobes, Simpson, & Berman, 2005), what I call "time-specific contingent treatment planning" with suicidal patients may not be suitable for every potential patient the clinician encounters (particularly those with cognitive disabilities, acute psychosis, or severe personality disorders). But clinicians have an obligation to transparently provide to any prospective patient (particularly if suicide is in the picture) a very clear message about what in their professional opinion is a reasonable plan for clinically proceeding, always with a focus on pursuing care that is in the patient's best interest. Whether the patient-"consumer" agrees and chooses to "buy" this treatment should be up to the patient-consumer, with no latent threat or clinical arm-twisting. As an aside let me note that even though I am not an enthusiast of coercive approaches to clinically preventing suicide, I still believe that there are times when suicidal patients should absolutely be hospitalized, even against their will. As previously noted, I always follow and comply with any and all legal statutes that require me to hospitalize a patient who poses a *clear and imminent* danger to self or others. But short of this most dire presentation, I am ardent about conducting reasonable negotiations with the patient that are designed to buy crucial time and trust, thereby creating a stronger alliance and that in turn may increase the patient's motivation to fight for his or her life.

Let me conclude this particular clinical and philosophical discourse by underscoring something quite literal and central to the CAMS approach to suicidality. The book you are reading is about the Collaborative Assessment and *Management* of Suicidality. CAMS is not CATS; I specifically decided that this clinical approach should emphasize the word *management* versus *treatment* in relation to dealing with suicidal risk. Clearly there are many treatment implications throughout this book, particularly in the course of this chapter on treatment planning. But the emphasis in CAMS is always on clinically managing the potential for suicide, until the patient has been fully "won over" to the side of wanting to live. CAMS care succeeds when patients ultimately conclude that they no longer *need* suicide as an option for coping with pain and suffering. The truth is that suicidal people only really give up on suicide when the purpose and value of suicide in their lives becomes obsolete, not because we have told them they cannot have it. Systematically helping to render suicide obsolete in the patient's life is a central goal in CAMS.

Clinical Treatment Planning in the Face of "Suicidal Blackmail"

A common struggle that clinicians often have with suicidal patients is the fear that if they do not accommodate or bend over backwards for the patient, the patient may attempt suicide or actually die by suicide. I refer to this as a form of "suicidal blackmail" within the clinical relationship. These cases may actually start out unremarkably only to later escalate into a situation in which the clinician becomes the paralyzed deer in the suicidal headlights of the patient. In other cases the potential struggle is obvious from the start. Invariably in these situations, the clinician ends up fielding phone calls at all hours, changing clinical practices, modifying boundaries, often spending inordinate amounts of time on a single, terrifying case. I know about this kind of struggle firsthand.

Even an otherwise erstwhile and conscientious clinician can lose perspective in the face of an escalating suicidal risk. In dealing with the risk, clinicians may feel compelled to do things that feel uncomfortable, to bend their rules and modify their usual and customary practice. Before they know it, the treatment is off the tracks and may career out of control. Treatments of this variety become increasingly reactive and chaotic—think of the little Dutch boy racing around trying to plug the leaks in the dike. More critically, however, is that such treatments are rarely ever in the patient's best interest. In addition, such frantic treatments often burn out competent and conscientious clinicians, leaving them miserable and feeling incompetent. All these various concerns and considerations have led to the fairly structured, transparent, and forthright approach that is seen in CAMS.

Among my arguments in relation to this topic is a contention that *not* being in clinical treatment is an obvious consideration for the suicidal patient, which is often overlooked as a genuine option by the patient and clinician alike. While I know this may be clinical heresy to some, I remain steadfast on this point and singularly focused on maximizing the potential for positive therapeutic outcomes. What I know from direct clinical experience and empirical research is that for treatment to work, the patient must be properly motivated and willing to proceed with the clinician in good faith. For the patient to be able to get motivated in a good-faith manner the clinician must create a clear transparent framework for how the work will proceed so the patient can make an informed choice about moving ahead.

I think any clinician working with a suicidal person (in particular) must be entirely clear about what he or she is planning on doing with the patient and why.

It is our job to form a professional opinion about what is in the patient's best interest and communicate that clearly to the patient. A treatment plan that best suits the patient's particular set of issues should be plainly presented to the patient so that an informed decision about engaging in that treatment can be made. Frankly, this process should happen whether suicide is in the picture or not. However if suicide is a consideration, my position is that it must be directly and squarely addressed as *the* primary clinical concern. We must have a direct and clear understanding with the patient about how we are going to deal with the threat of suicide. In this regard, I am rather rigid—certain conditions must be established for me to proceed with a suicidal patient in good faith. The patient, in turn, can then decide how to proceed—or not—in response to my professional judgment and my conditions for care.

As an example, let us consider an especially contentious issue that may arise between a clinician and the suicidal patient. Imagine a scenario in which a highly suicidal patient is seeking treatment and acknowledges ready access to a firearm in the home. In the course of discussing this access, the patient makes it known that he or she will not remove this weapon from the home environment at the request of the clinician, even for a relatively short-term period (e.g., a month). This standoff is difficult. On the one hand the patient may legitimately own a firearm. On the other hand, surveillance data from the Centers of Disease Control and other researchers have shown the clear lethal threat of a firearm in the home. As the clinician, I can gamble and acquiesce to the patient's refusal. Alternatively, I can make this issue a "deal breaker," and tell the patient I do not feel comfortable proceeding with care in the face of the risk posed by the weapon and the patient's refusal to remove it for the period of time in which we will pursue treatment. I choose to interpret the patient's refusal as therapeutic bad faith. In my view, such a position on the patient's part is a direct threat to our treatment plan, fundamentally undermining our treatment efforts to preserve life. Furthermore, I may be compelled to terminate the case and refer the patient on to another provider. This is not a political issue, but it is a clinical judgment issue. I am not saying a patient of mine may not own a firearm; rather, I am saying for the period of time that we have contracted to work on the issue of suicide, I reserve the right to assert a basic ground rule in order for therapy to proceed.

At this juncture, it is important to address legitimate concerns about the ethical issue of clinical "abandonment." The central ethical concern about abandonment centers on any unilateral action by the clinician of suddenly discontinuing clinical care, leaving the patient in a lurch. In cases of clinical abandonment, the patient has been suddenly dropped from clinical care in an unexpected manner leaving the patient vulnerable with no effort extended by the clinician to ensure that he or she receives any ongoing therapeutic care or support. It is a different situation when a clinician takes a thoughtful and principled position on behalf of the patient's best interest that may ultimately compel the clinician to bring the treatment to an end. In cases in which a patient's abject refusal to abide by certain necessary conditions of appropriate treatment compel the clinician to potentially bring the care to an end, it is important to (1) transparently work in the best interest of the patient, (2) be absolutely clear about the necessary elements of treatment (and why they are necessary), (3) make every reasonable effort to make referrals that would bridge the patient to other appropriate care, (4) seek professional consultation, and (5) carefully document one's decision making in relation to the patient's best interest (it is also wise to document in detail the input of one's professional consultant).

Consider the following case example. Some years ago a senior colleague of mine sought consultation on a particularly difficult case. I was quite familiar with this complex case from previous consultations. My colleague had been seeing this woman for almost 3 years; she was diagnosed with dysthymic disorder and borderline personality disorder. The treatment had been notably stormy and contentious with ongoing threats of suicide, two overdose attempts, and one psychiatric hospitalization. The situation that compelled him to seek me out yet again involved a new wrinkle in their embattled treatment relationship. The patient announced after missing a week of sessions (she was seen twice a week) that she had fired her psychiatrist and was now seeing a new psychiatrist who was completely changing her extensive medication regime. My colleague, a clinical psychologist by training, was shocked by the sudden development and insisted that she sign a release for him to make contact with the new psychiatrist. The patient refused, insisting that she did not want him talking to her new psychiatrist and she insisted that the new doctor was fine with this arrangement. My colleague explained that standard professional practice and ethics required a coordinated clinical effort and that his inability to consult with the other member of her treatment team was not in her best interest and this new arrangement was ultimately unacceptable to him. She would not budge; in fact, he noted that she appeared to "enjoy" defying him in this manner. After discussing the history of the case, the ethics, his counntertransference, and various other issues, we concluded that he had to take a strong position that his work with her would need to come to an end if she was unwilling to let him coordinate her care with the physician. He reasonably gave her 3 weeks to change her mind. But at the end of 3 weeks, she remained steadfast and their tumultuous work together came to a necessary end. In their final session he reviewed the basis for this course of action and offered to refer her to other providers. He was even willing to take her back if she changed her mind. However, she did not change her mind, and she left in an angry snit announcing that she would be seeing her psychiatrist for both her medicine and her psychotherapy. While this case example is not particularly satisfying from an outcome standpoint, I believe my colleague had little choice and that he proceeded in a completely ethical and appropriate manner in bringing this case to a necessary close.

The point in all this is that it is crucial to know and assert one's clinical judgment about how certain aspects of the treatment *must* proceed. When working with a patient who refuses to meet certain necessary conditions of treatment, I have said, for example,

> ". . . Your position that you reserve the right to kill yourself during your treatment is untenable to me; it simply won't work for us to proceed in that fashion. To that end, you may need to find another therapist—which I will of course help you do—or maybe you should reconsider your overall readiness to engage in psychotherapy at all. . . ."

Clinicians in my workshops are often shocked by my taking this kind of position with the patient. In response, I clarify that I am not trying to use a paradoxical intervention or be provocative with the patient. I am simply being clear about my limits and the constraints of the treatment that I am able and willing to offer and why this is so. I always recommend to suicidal patients that they should seriously consider engaging in a clinical treatment that endeavors to pursue their best interest *before* exercising the more dire option of suicide. But if they are to be in treatment with me, I want them to be fully in treatment; not ready to jump out of the "treatment car" while it is moving.

It is therefore important to be transparent about the process of the clinical engagement, to develop treatment plans and contracts carefully, and to work within finite specific time frames. We cannot let the patient's problems, suicidal threats, or Axis II pathology be the "tail that wags the dog" of the treatment. Letting that happen is never in the patient's best interest.

This discussion returns us to the importance of negotiating relatively short, good-faith, time-specific, suicide-relevant treatment contracts. Critically, at the end of each treatment contract period a mutual discussion ensues as to whether we should clinically proceed. Invariably someone at my workshop will ask, "What happens if you take this rigid approach and tell the patient that she is not ready for therapy because she refuses one of your conditions . . . and then she proceeds to go home and kill herself that very evening. Aren't you liable?"

Such a scenario would undoubtedly be a tragedy and I would feel horrible. But frankly such a prospect comes with the territory and can happen with any suicidal person, regardless of whether one uses the approach I am advocating or not. It is a risk we all face. However, regardless of whether I suggested that the patient was a poor candidate for treatment (e.g., by virtue of refusing to comply with a key treatment condition), the determination of liability will rest on one critical hindsight question: Was the patient at the moment he or she left my office in clear and imminent danger? If the answer is yes, that person should have been sent to the hospital—voluntarily or involuntarily if necessary—to ensure that the person does not perform a self-harm behavior. A failure to effect a hospitalization under these circumstances may well make the clinician liable. But if the answer is no, we have a tragic situation to be sure, but nevertheless a situation in which a prospective patient was neither able nor willing to accept a reasonable time-limited treatment proposal that was designed to save the patient's life. There are no guarantees that one will not be sued in such a scenario, and I am always impressed by the willingness of plaintiff attorneys to explore malpractice even in extremely weak cases. But one must be clear about their usual and customary practice—why they made the decisions they made and how they must always loop back to what was in their patient's best interest. If this position can be further bolstered by theory or data it is even more defendable in a hindsight situation. As will be noted repeatedly in Chapter 8, the role of detailed and thorough documentation is key in relation to the "Monday-morning quarterbacking" that invariably occurs in malpractice cases where the wisdom of hindsight is plain.

Experience has demonstrated to me that the alternative to my way of thinking is simply indefensible—that a clinician would knowingly begin (or continue) a therapeutic relationship with a patient giving up on critical and necessary conditions of treatment. It is metaphorically akin to knowingly embarking (or continuing) on a potentially dangerous boat trip with the suicidal patient in spite of a rather large hole in the bow of the vessel—it is a lose–lose scenario for the clinician and the patient. If, however, a clinician acquiesces on basic conditions of appropriate care, it is akin to saying to the patient that it is acceptable to be unreasonable (i.e., it is okay to not meet the clinician halfway in good faith to pursue a reasonable time-specific treatment that is designed to save the patient's life). Like many of you reading this book, I have been there and done that. Such an approach does not work for the patient and it certainly does not work for the clinician. Such acquiescence on the part of clinician in the face of suicidal blackmail is not in the best interest of the patient and I cannot abide it.

CAMS OUTPATIENT TREATMENT PLANNING: SECTION C OF THE SSF

Having now addressed the philosophical and conceptual underpinnings of the CAMS approach to treatment planning, let us now shift to more concrete procedural considerations. To briefly review, in the last chapter we left off with the completion of Section B of the SSF suicide risk assessment. As discussed, we have typically spent roughly a half hour in session working collaboratively with the patient completing Sections A and B of the SSF. Completion of the SSF risk assessment is a critical juncture in the CAMS index session, it is the point at which clinical attention shifts to collaboratively developing an outpatient treatment plan. The CAMS approach to outpatient treatment planning was fundamentally shaped by the thinking of several leading figures in the field—particularly Aaron Beck (1986), David Rudd (Rudd et al., 2001), Marsha Linehan (1993a, 1993b, 2005), and Edwin Shneidman (1993, 1998).

Overview to Negotiating the Treatment Plan

What follows are key elements that I believe should guide any clinical negotiation of a patient's safety:

- The clinician should be absolutely clear to the patient in relation to legal statutes pertaining to confidentiality and imminent danger to self—which should be handled in relation to informed consent forms that should be read and completed *prior* to direct clinical contact.
- The clinician should emphasize with the patient the importance of mutual give and take—there are reasonable expectations that each party can have of the other.
- The clinician should communicate empathy of the patient's suicidal wish— appreciating the patient's feeling that suicide may be a tempting means for dealing with *seemingly* unbearable pain.
- However, the clinician should always ask the patient the following question: Is suicide in fact the *best* way to cope?
- The clinician should always negotiate in relation to time-based considerations and persist in exploring all possibilities for *delaying* suicidal behavior.
- The clinician should fundamentally seek a reasonable, good-faith, time-specific, agreement with the patient to give treatment a fair chance of making a difference.
- The clinician should be clear that the patient's suicide-specific treatment plan will focus on (1) increasing the patient's psychological pain tolerance, (2) creating alternative and better ways for the patient to cope with psychological pain, and (3) working to ultimately make the patient's life worth living.

Guided by these considerations, the clinician and patient are in a pivotal position to negotiate a reasonable and viable suicide-specific outpatient treatment plan. As previously discussed, within CAMS there is an overt emphasis on the development of a viable treatment plan during the index session, which by its nature will justify outpatient care. The crucial message to the patient is that we are interested in keeping them *out* of the hospital if at all possible. I typically introduce SSF Section C by saying the following:

> "Now we need to work on the treatment plan. To do this we need to fully consider all the information we have learned about your pain and suffering and overall risk for suicide. To make an effective plan, we may need to refer back to Sections A and B of the assessment we just did to develop some specific goals and targets of our treatment. Since we must take the issue of suicide very seriously, our first consideration is how are we going to deal with your suicide risk potential? To this end, I want to be clear that my goal is to find a way to keep you out of the hospital. However, for us to achieve the goal of keeping you out of the hospital, we must develop a viable outpatient treatment plan that we are both comfortable with and that we are both committed to . . ."

In specific reference to SSF Section C (Appendix A), we see that the treatment planning portion of the form is organized into the following four sections: (1) Problem # and Problem Description, (2) Goals and Objectives (and Evidence for Attainment), (3) Intervention (Time and Frequency), and (4) Estimated Number of Sessions. These sections are to be completed by the clinician in consultation with the patient—in this sense the patient serves as a *coauthor* of the treatment plan. It is important to underscore that within Section C of the SSF, Problem 1 (Self-Harm Potential) is *not* negotiable. Eliminating self-harm potential is the number-one goal within CAMS. Similarly, the Goal and Objective of "Outpatient Safety" is also not negotiable. How the problem of self-harm potential and the goal of outpatient safety are collaboratively addressed in relation to specific clinical interventions is the crux of CAMS outpatient treatment planning. At the heart of this particular suicide-specific treatment planning endeavor is the Crisis Response Plan.

Problem 1: Negotiating the Crisis Response Plan in CAMS

Following recent work in the field—most notably by David Rudd (e.g., Rudd, Mandrusiak, & Joiner, 2006)—the CAMS approach to treatment planning emphatically eschews the widespread use of "safety contracts," otherwise called "no-suicide contracts" (Jobes & Drozd, 2004). In truth, safety/no-suicide contracts are neither contractual (in any legal sense) nor really about ensuring patient safety. In its widespread contemporary use, safety contracting tends to be a somewhat coercive process of extracting from suicidal patients a verbal or written promise of what they *won't* do if they feel suicidal. Failure to obtain such a promise from patients necessarily prompts an inpatient hospitalization. Like Rudd, a growing number of contemporary clinical suicidologists, are increasingly critical of the standard use of these contracts as being fundamentally flawed (Ellis, 2004; Jobes, 2004b; Linehan, 1993a). Along with my colleagues, I have seen dozens of malpractice cases where the clinician naively believes that a no-suicide contract is truly protective in terms of malpractice liability. But invariably these contracts come back to haunt the clinician, *because the contract obviously failed!*

As an alternative to safety/no-suicide contracts, Rudd and colleagues (2001, 2006) have argued that clinicians should work to develop outpatient treatment plans that emphasize what patients *will* do if they feel impulsive, lonely, upset, or suicidal, versus what they *won't* do. To this end, Rudd and colleagues advocate the development and use of a Crisis Response Plan. This progressive approach to suicide-specific treatment planning has been directly imported into how a CAMS clinician negotiates the treatment plan with the suicidal patient as it is recorded within Section C of the SSF under the heading "Crisis Response Plan." Thus, a Crisis Response Plan is always negotiated in direct response to Problem 1 (Self-Harm Potential), in order to meet the central Goal/Objective of clinical care (Outpatient Safety).

CAMS encourages the initiation of clinician and patient negotiations about the specific management of suicidal impulses as well as the overall maintenance of outpatient safety and stability. These negotiations emphasize a good-faith commitment by *both* parties to earnestly engage in a plan of active clinical work for a mutually agreed period of time. Closely linked to these negotiations are a series of concrete strategic safety interventions that are designed to decrease the immediate dangerousness of the situation and provide structure and support should future crisis situations arise. What follows are various specific concrete safety interventions to consider for a typical CAMS treatment plan.

Negotiating Clinical Contact

The relative "dose" of clinical contact between patient and clinician is always a crucial consideration in outpatient treatment planning with suicidal patients. Generally speaking, it is widely recognized that, at least in the short term, more contact with a suicidal patient is often appropriate (Berman et al., 2006; Maris, Berman, & Silverman, 2000). Typically, this means scheduling more frequent meetings than once per week—usually twice a week sometimes even three times a week during the most acute phase of risk. As discussed further on, clinical contact is not limited to face-to-face meetings. Phone calls and possibly e-mails represent viable alternative tools for making and maintaining between-session contacts. The "right" amount of clinical contact is often a difficult call. Finding the right balance of clinical contact can be challenging—too much contact can become behaviorally reinforcing, leading to an overdependence on the clinician, a desire for even more contact with the clinician, and may potentially undermine any efforts for the patient to learn to cope by using self-soothing techniques. On the other hand, too little contact and access can reinforce the sense of isolation that often plagues suicidal patients. It is crucial to talk directly to the patient about the amount of contact that is needed; by engaging the patient in this discussion it becomes a joint effort to find the elusive "right" balance.

Removing Access to the Means

I have already spoken about the importance of the patient's removing access to lethal means in the living environment. This treatment condition is particularly relevant in the case of an obviously available lethal means, such as firearms—the number-one choice of both male and female completers in the United States across all ages (National Center for Health Statistics, 2003). But removing access to lethal means also applies to a stash of lethal medications, a rope that has been put aside for hanging, or even razor blades to be used for cutting. Obviously, there are limits to this intervention. For someone who entertains carbon monoxide poisoning using the car and the home garage, it is unrealistic to have the patient turn in the car keys or to lock the patient out of the garage. Similarly, someone living in a high-rise apartment building with serious potential for lethal jumping cannot be realistically asked to move, although I did have a patient who was repeatedly tempted to jump from her 11th-story apartment stay at her girl-friend's basement apartment during high-risk periods. Eventually this chronically suicidal patient's lethal means was removed by having her apartment windows and balcony door permanently sealed by her carpenter boyfriend to literally block her ability to jump, which promptly removed the temptation.

One particular case during my clinical internship year made an indelible impression on me in relation to removing access to lethal means. In my first rotation in the mental hygiene clinic, I began seeing a former Navy SEAL veteran who had several grievances against the military for egregious medical care. For example, a military-related injury on a submarine required a surgical procedure on his right knee, yet the procedure was performed on his uninjured *left* knee! Not only did the surgeon operate on the incorrect knee, the surgery itself was botched, leaving his formerly healthy left knee in worse condition than his still injured right knee. Unfortunately, there were actually a couple of additional bungled medical procedures that occurred before he was ultimately medically discharged from the Navy. Beyond these horrific medical experiences in the military, my patient was also having problems with the VA in terms of receiving a service connection to compensate for his service-related injuries. Not surprisingly, he was seeing me due to psychological stress, anxiety, depression, and self-esteem problems.

Among the various issues, a particularly disturbing concern was that the patient had a recurring dream in which he would march up to Capitol Hill in Washington, D.C., and find himself surrounded by his U.S. senators and his congressional representative. In the dream, as his elected officials assembled around him on the steps of the Capitol, he would take out his handgun and shoot himself in the head. The patient vehemently denied any suicidal thoughts, had no suicidal history, and was genuinely puzzled and alarmed by this dream. At the time I truly believed the patient when he said he was not suicidal. Nevertheless, my clinical supervisor for this case wisely encouraged me to ask the patient to remove his handgun from his home during our treatment. With some trepidation I asked the patient to give up his gun for the time being. Much to my relief he readily agreed and gave the gun to his father for safekeeping.

Eleven months later my patient—shamefaced—came in for a Monday morning session. He reported to me that he had just been through the most difficult weekend of his life. The patient had been fired on Friday evening from his job as a real estate agent because he was having difficulty getting around to various properties due to his knee injuries (and he refused to use crutches). The next morning, my patient fought with his girlfriend, which resulted in a breakup. Feeling despondent and miserable over the course of the day, he went to a bar on Saturday night and got extremely intoxicated. By the evening's end, he headed home determined to take his life. In his drunken state, he made his way to the dresser to find his gun with the intent to shoot himself and thereby end his misery. But the gun was not there because he had turned over the firearm to his father almost a year ago at my request. When the patient woke up the following morning with a miserable hangover, he contemplated what might have happened if that gun had been sitting in his dresser drawer that night. To me it was an incredible lesson. It was an element of our treatment plan that at the time seemed like too much to ask and not really necessary, yet it may well have been a life-saving intervention.

I know there can be some uncertainty about how exactly we get the patient to remove access to lethal means. For example, I once had a senior colleague with a locked file drawer stuffed full of confiscated bottles of pills, clips of bullets, razors, ropes, and gun lock keys. He even had a couple of dismantled pistols he had collected from some suicidal patients. I personally do not collect such items and I do not recommend this approach because of my discomfort about having weapons brought into the office. But my colleague was comfortable with this approach and his track record of seeing suicidal patients was quite impressive. I personally prefer to put some measure of trust in the patient and I usually make some arrangement with the patient to get some form of third-party verification that the means are in fact secured, increasing the safety of the living environment.

Clarifying Between-Session Access: The Coping Card

Probably one of the most important potential interventions in working with suicidal patients involves emergency access that the patient has to reach a clinician
between sessions. The clinician's between-session availability in case of emergency is complex because of fundamental boundary issues whenever a patient
contacts a clinician who is "off the clock." Moreover, there are significant implications in relation to potential liability in malpractice scenarios. In relation to
this latter concern, it is very important for clinicians to clearly think through
how they want to handle between-session emergency access. They must clearly
establish their "usual and customary practice" in relation to this important topic
because they will need to be able to defend how they handle emergency availability. In a malpractice scenario a question may be whether the clinician devi-
ated from his or her usual and customary practice related to emergency access.
In turn, the clinician must be able to defend the usual and customary practice
that was used in relation to the "standard of care" (which is discussed in depth
in Chapter 8).

Standard of care in terms of patient access is frankly hard to know. I have personally seen a broad range of ways in which clinicians handle this particular
issue. For example, some may offer 9-to-5 availability and have the patient use a
crisis hotline after hours and on weekends. Others may give out their personal
cell phone number or their beeper number, being virtually available 24/7. The
exact best practice in relation to emergency access is difficult to know and the protection of the clinician's personal and professional life from patients who may
abuse this emergency access is an important consideration.

I have found the use of a "Crisis Card" to be an effective solution to the issue
of emergency access. In the cognitive therapy tradition, Aaron Beck and colleagues first developed the use of coping cards that prompt different strategies
for the patient to deal with problematic thoughts and feelings (Beck, Rush, Shaw,
& Emery, 1979). In addition to Beck, others have made valuable contributions in
relation to using this kind of concrete strategy (Chiles & Strosahl, 1995; Linehan,
1993a; Rudd et al., 2001).

Generally speaking, the Crisis Card strategy fits nicely into the CAMS philosophy of collaborative empowerment of the patient. Specifically, in the course of
treatment planning, it is important that the patient know that there is a reliable
approach to cope with a difficult situation should an emergency situation arise
between sessions. Typically in the course of this discussion, I take out my business card, flip it over, write "Crisis Card" at the center top, and then mark down
the left side of the card the numbers 1, 2, 3, 4, and 5. I then propose that we come
up with five things that the patient can do if a crisis situation occurs. Ideally these
ideas come from the patient and must be protherapeutic, typically involving

behavioral activation. For example, going out and getting drunk is not an acceptable item for the coping card. Alternatively, activities such as exercising, therapeutic writing, or talking to a supportive friend are all excellent examples of coping ideas. Ideally, these items come from the patient, but I do chime in with suggestions if the patient is stuck. The following is a list of protherapeutic Crisis Card items used by suicidal patients of mine:

- Going for a walk
- Writing in my journal
- Taking a nice, hot bath
- Doing my nails
- Walking my dog
- Listening to music
- E-mailing a supportive friend
- Taking a nap
- Doing some artwork
- Reading one of my therapeutic books

- Brushing out my hair 100 times
- Going to church to pray
- Meditating
- Playing on my Gameboy
- Reading a magazine
- Watching the Animal Planet channel on TV
- Writing a letter to an old friend

This list represents the type of activities that one looks for on the Crisis Card—protherapeutic activities that engage, redirect, and behaviorally activate the patient. Critically, after the process of developing five activities to put on the card, I rather ceremoniously take the card and add a sixth item: an emergency phone number where the patient can receive direct clinical care. In my own case, this is my business line phone number at home. For those working in an agency with coverage or hospital centers this number would be the emergency coverage number. Whatever the case, there should be a way that the suicidal patient can access a clinician in the event of a true emergency. Again in my own case, in a life-threatening crisis, I want the patient to call my home business line after hours—which is separate from the family phone line, which is unlisted. For obvious reasons, I do not want my wife or my children answering a patient's crisis call. In relation to this topic, I say to the patient something along the lines of:

"Okay, this is your Crisis Card. Your commitment to me and to your overall treatment is that you will do each item on this card should you find yourself in a crisis state—feeling impulsive, really upset, or suicidal. The goal here is for you to learn to cope in different ways than you are used to and to develop ways of getting out of trouble on your own. If you do each of these items on the card and you are still in a bad state, then you call me at this number, which is my home business line. If I do not answer, leave me a message and I will typically get back to you within the hour. If you still need to talk to someone, you can call the hotline number I gave you, but I will be calling you back soon if you leave me a message. The point is that I am interested in being available to you if you are in a true emergency crisis state. You will know that the situation is a true emergency by virtue of having gone through all five ways of coping and you feel that you are still in serious trouble. To be clear, you are only to call me after you have done the five preceding coping ideas, if none of those seems to work, then you know to call me."

The beauty of this Crisis Card approach is that it clearly communicates a crucial therapeutic message to the patient: *You* can learn to cope with your crises; if that does not work, I will endeavor to be directly available to you for true emergency support. Rudd and colleagues (2001) conceptualize this as self-regulation training—the first five Crisis Card items are designed to improve the patient's *internal* resources to manage a crisis before turning to *external resources*—direct engagement of the clinician. The treatment idea here emphasizes the importance of the patient developing a "thicker psychological skin," to better withstand the ups and downs of life—the disappointments, the hurts, and injuries that happen to all of us. Using the Crisis Card as I just described is an excellent way for the patient to learn about developing a thicker mental skin.

When I discuss the use of Crisis Cards at my workshops I am often asked whether patients actually use this card as I just described—what is to stop them from skipping 1–5 and going right to calling me at home? In response, I note that the vast majority of patients do use the Crisis Card appropriately. Although all patients may not use it perfectly, most catch on to the intent of what the Crisis Card is meant to be, which in part is to help clarify for the patient what *is* a mental health emergency, and what is not. In more than 15 years of practice I have only been forced to change my unlisted number at home twice, not an inordinate number given the number of suicidal patients I have worked with over these years. As an aside, it has been helpful for my patients to know that I have a dedicated home line for professional purposes so that neither they nor my family will be put in an awkward position.

The Crisis Card has been highly effective for many of my patients, often in different and unexpected ways. For example, many years ago I worked with a patient who simply took out the card and looked at the items, which made her feel better—she did not do any of the coping items, just looking at the card was all she needed. Another example involves a teenage patient whose eyes filled with tears when we completed the card. She could not believe that I cared so much that I was willing to give my number at home. Another successful Crisis Card case was of a patient who was completely skeptical about using the approach. The weekend following our developing her Crisis Card was marked by a series of conflicts and disappointments. She warily took out her Crisis Card and began marching through each item, certain that this effort was a waste of time and that she would soon be calling me as the only option to resolve her crisis. This patient first took a walk, then had a long talk with her roommate—neither helped. In good faith she pursued item 3, which was to take a nap. She stretched out on her bed at 7:00 P.M. and much to her shock woke up the following morning at 7:00 A.M., a 12-hour nap! She could barely wait to tell me in our next session that the Crisis Card had worked exceptionally well—she had gotten through a tough night on her own when she was virtually certain that she was going to need to call me.

I am a committed advocate of the Crisis Card method. I would encourage the interested reader to read more on this compelling technique as discussed by David Rudd and colleagues (2001, 2006), Beck and colleagues (1979), and those who have worked in the dialectical behavior therapy tradition (e.g., Chiles & Strosahl, 1995). Various authors primarily in the cognitive-behavioral camp have made outstanding contributions in this particular area of intervention. For example, building off of Beck's work in reference to the "suicidal mode," David Rudd's use of the technique is a bit more elaborate and structured and also includes the use of an ER in extremely urgent situations (Rudd et al., 2006).

Developing a Hope Kit

Building again off the important work of Beck and colleagues (Brown, Hare, et al., 2005; Henriques, Beck, & Brown, 2003), there are additional concrete interventions that can be used during moments of crisis. One such approach is the "Hope Kit" developed by Beck's group. They think of this approach as a memory aid to help the suicidal patient recall why he or she should otherwise want to live. The use of the Hope Kit is embedded in a 10-session cognitive therapy treatment that has excellent empirical support for reducing suicide attempt behaviors (Brown, Hare, et al., 2005). The Hope Kit is constructed with the therapist's help and may involve simply taking a shoe box and filling it with life-affirming items and meaningful mementoes that instill a sense of hope such as pictures, trinkets, letters, awards, small pieces of artwork, and so on. Anything can be included that might remind the patient of why the struggle to live is worth fighting.

I have used this Hope Kit idea with a handful of patients with great success. For many years in my training workshops I have referred to the notion of the patient developing a better "psychological tool kit" as a compelling metaphor. The Hope Kit is an excellent concrete manifestation of this metaphor. Patients need resources, tools, and new ways of dealing with hard times. In the short term, at least these concrete cognitive-behavioral interventions can make a meaningful difference particularly in relation to helping patients see that they can help and soothe themselves.

Increasing Social Supports

It is well known in the suicide literature that social engagement and integration is a key to keeping a suicidal person safe. In fact, my colleague Thomas Joiner (2005) has built his entire theory of suicide around the central importance of social influences in relation to suicide. He argues that suicidal people are routinely plagued by two different, but important, social experiences: (1) that suicidal people often deeply perceive that they have become a burden on those who love them, and (2) that suicidal people often experience "thwarted belongingness"—that efforts to connect to others have failed or that they simply do not belong to a meaningful group of others. The antidote to these types of perceptions is clarification that the patient's loved ones care and will be there for the patient. While these patients may in fact be burdensome to friends and family, few survivors ever acknowledge being relieved or better off when their loved one takes his or her life. In other words, it is important to encourage—even push—a suicidal person to find meaningful attachments to others—this could be through a therapeutic group, through Alcoholics Anonymous (AA), or even by encouraging a budding interest in becoming a fan of a particular sports team. More typically, however, we are talking about the importance of developing a reliable support system and the need to guard the patient at risk from social isolation, particularly during periods of increased risk. In relation to these concerns, I am particularly supportive of patients adding virtually any form of interpersonal support to their Crisis Card.

Homo sapiens are relational creatures; we live in family units, tribes, villages, and cities. Like Joiner, I have asserted elsewhere (Jobes, 2000) that most suicides can almost always be linked to interpersonal issues. Clearly the absence—or presence—of certain key relationships can be suicidogenic. As I have repeatedly noted throughout this book, the relational component to CAMS is central to success. CAMS underscores the importance of working hard to advance and develop a strong clinical alliance with the patient in order to help the patient learn to cope more effectively with seemingly unbearable psychological pain and suffering. Bottom line, as clinicians we must do what we can to decrease the suicidal patient's social isolation.

Beyond purely clinical considerations, from a liability perspective the engagement of collateral social supports can prove to be quite protective (Wise et al., 2005). Leading plaintiff attorneys in malpractice wrongful death suicide cases assert that it is important to engage key significant others in the patient's treatment. They assert that clinicians should persevere to secure releases from the patient that enable the clinician to contact and engage key family members and relational supports in service of treatment and safety. I would contend that engagement of others is often an absolutely crucial move for the patient's stability and overall treatment. There are, however, case exceptions in which contacting significant others could prove to be a disaster that undermines working in the patient's best interest. Whatever the case, engaging others in the patient's care should be routinely considered. Cynically, these are the people who will be suing the clinician in a worse-case outcome. In this vein, I frankly suspect litigation is less likely if the suicide does not come from out of the blue and if family members were aware of or actually engaged in the patient's safety management plan. Less cynically, it just makes good clinical sense to engage family and friends as key supports—increasing the patient's sense of belongingness and eliminating any notion that loved ones will be better off without the patient.

Using the Full Range of Modalities

When considering the treatment plan in general, and the Crisis Response Plan in particular, it is important to use all possible relevant modalities. For example, all the obvious clinical modalities—group, couple, family therapies—should all be considered. Referral for psychiatric consultation should always be considered; in fact, failure to refer a patient for possible medication consultation can be cited as a specific complaint in relation to the standard of care. I think it is always important to be creative in treatment planning and to think inside *and* outside the box. This means thinking of all possible treatments and interventions, conventional and otherwise, within reason.

Increasing Behavioral Activation

In recent years I have been impressed with the evolving literature on behavioral activation (e.g., Jacobson, Martell, & Dimidjian, 2001). Although I know working with cognitions and affect is extremely important, the bottom-line ability for the patient to become *behaviorally* engaged in life is particularly crucial. To this end, we see the important role that behavioral activation plays in the Crisis Card approach to coping, discussed earlier in this section. I know there is a basic conundrum here. Most depressed and suicidal people feel behaviorally deactivated. The dilemma is that the antidote to their problem *is* their problem! People who are depressed and plagued with suicidal suffering routinely do not feel like going for a run or getting things on their "to do" list done. In many cases, simply getting out of bed seems like an insurmountable challenge. Yet, as clinicians we must do our best to light a fire under the patient to get the patient engaged in life. In this sense, I often spend a significant amount of time in session talking about physical exercise, making obtainable goals, or writing in a blank book for journaling. I am often impressed by how poor my patients are at planning and getting things done. They often describe an utter inability to plan at all and have no motivation to get things done. Accordingly, we often spend a great deal of time talking about reasonable to-do lists and how to successfully use a planner or an electronic device as a way to maintain a schedule and help patients meet their goals.

Often efforts on my part to introduce strategies related to planning and the systematic pursuit of reasonable goals are met with moans from the patient that he or she simply "can't." But I remain fairly persistent on this front. I whittle away at the patient's reluctance by breaking down the behavior goal into (sometimes comical) minigoals that even the most depressed patient will ultimately admit they can do. I once had an obese patient who insisted she could not exercise; the prospect was just too overwhelming for her to even consider. I insisted that we break down the goal and work toward successive approximations of the larger goal. Again she refused. When she refused to consider a 30-minute walk each day, I nevertheless persisted. Finally with mutual laughter we negotiated an agreement where she would commit to walking for 3 minutes each morning, which was only a little walk down her block. In the coming weeks we increased the walking by 5-minute increments until she reached a point where she voluntarily felt comfortable increasing her walking regiment on her own. In 2 years she was up to walking twice a day for 45 minutes and had lost 60 pounds, taking great pride in her success. She had a new sense of self-discipline, enjoyed the exercise, and was very pleased about her weight loss. I love this example because it underscores that behavioral activation can always be pursued in an incremental fashion with good-faith negotiations, persistence, patience, and supportive understanding.

Creating Future Linkage

As discussed in Chapter 2, we have conducted SSF research that underscores the importance of future thinking and the development of plans, goals, and hope for the future as potentially protective buffer against suicidality. Current research in this area is quite promising. The work of Mark Williams (2001) related to future thinking and Aaron Beck's (Beck & Steer, 1988) work on the importance of developing hope in the face of hopelessness are two examples of important innovations in this area. These researchers, among others, are making clear that future thinking is a key assessment for suicidal risk as well as a point of clinical intervention with suicidal patients (see also O'Connor, O'Connor, O'Connor, Smallwood, & Miles, 2004).

My own research is increasingly targeting the importance of future thinking as an assessment and intervention focus for suicidality (Jobes, 2004b). The point is that suicidal people invariably feel that the future holds no promise for them. This is a potentially deadly preoccupation that we as clinicians must directly confront with the patient. Future thinking and the ability to better plan and foster hope are central to helping tip the balance from a preoccupation with reasons for dying to reasons for living. As clinicians we should be unabashed in our active pursuit of reasons for living in the patient's life. I often reflect that as a career suicidologist I have spent a great deal of time trying to understand why suicidal people want to die. However, the more I study suicide the more focused I am about what it means to be alive. SSF data discussed earlier (Jobes et al., 2004) clearly show that what makes the "world go round" in the land of the living are our plans, hopes, and goals for the future that tend to focus on our relationships, our work, and our sense of self in the world. These are the elements of life that we all aspire to pursue. In the case of suicidal people, they have either lost track of these foci in life or never had them in the first place. Our job is to see that we do our best to help them see that they may be able to recover these essential life elements or perhaps discover them for the first time.

Problems 2 and 3

While the number-one problem to be addressed in CAMS is self-harm potential, this focus does not preclude consideration of other significant problems thereafter. Inevitably these problems are almost always linked to the issue of suicide anyway. The collaborative completion of SSF Sections A and B usually identifies themes of problems, particularly through the qualitative SSF assessments. It is often true that a certain issue, relationship, or problem will appear across the various SSF assessments that usually indicate at least two other specific targets to be addressed by the treatment plan. Sometimes these are symptoms of psychopathology, which prompts diagnosis-specific interventions of various durations. For example, depression is often identified as a specific treatment problem prompting interventions that range from medication consultation to specific psychosocial treatments for depression. Many times problems are focused on a relationship or vocational struggle prompting interventions such as couple therapy or perhaps specific vocational assessment or counseling. Again, I am not trying to dictate the kinds of problems to be addressed or the best treatments or theoretical orientation to address them. I am simply noting that the SSF Section C for treatment planning can accommodate additional issues that can be easily incorporated into the patient's CAMS outpatient treatment plan.

Commitment to Treatment

SSF Section C is completed by two final dichotomously stated (yes or no) assessments: (1) whether the patient understands and commits to the outpatient treatment plan, and (2) whether the patient is in clear and imminent danger. These two items represent a clinical and medicolegal bottom line. If patients commit to their treatment *and* are not in imminent danger, they may proceed with a sense of treatment direction, focus, and a clear understanding—through the Crisis Response Plan—of what to do should they find themselves in an emergent crisis.

Again, Rudd and colleagues (2001, 2006) have written compellingly about working with the suicidal patient to commit to the treatment process. Within their "Commitment to Treatment" approach there is a written statement that highlights seven points of committing to all aspects of the treatment process, including the following:

1. Attending sessions.
2. Setting goals.
3. Voicing my opinions, thoughts, and feelings honestly and openly with my therapist.
4. Being actively involved during sessions.
5. Completing homework assignments.
6. Experimenting with new behaviors and new ways of doing things.
7. Implementing my crisis response plan when needed.

Refer to Rudd and colleagues (2001) for a more detailed discussion of their approach to treating suicidal behavior. These authors have written an exceptionally thoughtful book in the cognitive-behavioral tradition with useful suggestions about crisis intervention with suicidal cases and valuable ways of thinking about treatment. In many respects, the structure and focus of their cognitive-behavioral approach lends itself well to working with suicidal patients, particularly in the earliest phases of care. However, there are still many other approaches (refer to Berman et al., 2006, for a review), including psychodynamic approaches, that are quite viable, particularly if a longer-term treatment is possible (e.g., Jobes, 1995b; Jobes & Karmel, 1996).

Whatever theoretical approach the clinician chooses to embrace, within CAMS the initial treatment planning goal in the index session is always the same. We are looking for a sense that we can in fact proceed reasonably with the suicidal patient by virtue of work done in the index session completing SSF Sections A–C. Experience has shown, that when we have gone through the collaborative process of CAMS assessment and outpatient treatment planning we should have a very clear sense as to whether the patient is truly on board—committed to care and willing to fight for his or her life. If not, an inpatient psychiatric hospitalization may well be the necessary intervention. However, if the case is able to proceed on an outpatient basis, I recommend giving the patient a photocopy of the first two pages of the SSF. I find that patients appreciate having the documents to take home; they end up reflecting on the assessment further and they also find value in referring to their treatment plan. The notion of transparency is crucial to

CAMS—I do not want all this assessment and treatment planning to be mysterious to the patient; I want the patient directly involved, understanding where we have been and where we are going.

The Air Force Case Example: The Treatment Plan

Having now thoroughly reviewed the elements of CAMS-based treatment planning in Section C of the SSF, let us reconsider the previously discussed case of the suicidal airman. As shown in Figure 4.2, a detailed treatment plan was developed in this case. The clinician negotiated a reasonable Crisis Response Plan that included "the development of a safety action plan." In this case the "action plan" involved engaging the patient's first sergeant and commanding officer, to let them know how depressed the patient had been over his assignment to security forces (something he was explicitly promised at recruitment he would not have to do). There was also some discussion about having the patient reassigned for a couple of weeks away from the night shift in the guard booth and temporary removal of his firearm. Ultimately, the commanding officer indicated that cross-training was possible within the next 4 months, which would enable the patient to get a new job in computers. The action plan also included pairing the patient up with some of his buddies in the unit for added support to "do some fun activities with the guys." The clinician and patient also developed a Crisis Card together, which the patient was actually enthusiastic to use should he get into trouble. The level of patient engagement—even enthusiasm—related to dealing with the problem of "self-harm potential" was obvious to the clinician. They were able to work out a reasonable Crisis Response Plan for a 2-week period that would include twice-a-week meetings. With this intervention in place the clinician felt comfortable pushing hospitalization on to the backburner (a decision that greatly relieved the patient, who did not want to have to be locked up in the "looney bin").

In terms of additional problems, the clinician and patient agreed that some focus should be brought to bear on the patient's depression. Accordingly, they agreed to have the patient see the center psychiatrist for possible antidepressant medication. In addition, the clinician would provide standard cognitive-behavioral psychotherapy over the course of eight treatment sessions. The clinician and patient also agreed that an intervention with the marriage was clearly warranted. The clinician perceived significant problems in the couple's communications and developed a couple therapy intervention for four sessions.

As I have elsewhere described (Jobes & Drozd, 2004), the outcome of this case was outstanding. The patient was almost immediately buoyed by the response of his supervisors and friends who were more than willing to support him in the midst of his crisis. His wife, who was initially wary, quickly got on board the therapeutic bandwagon as they made notable progress in couple meetings. The patient had a clear therapeutic response in relation to the combination of Prozac and the cognitive-behavioral therapy. Bottom line, suicidal thinking was completely extinguished in 5 sessions; overall symptom distress was significantly reduced after 10 sessions. The case was successfully terminated after the 11th session. Although not all cases will have such a dramatic and robust outcome, one must remember that only 2 months prior to terminating the CAMS treatment, this troubled patient had been sitting in a guard booth late at night on the outskirts of the base with a gun in his mouth praying to God for the strength to pull the trigger. Obviously this case is an excellent example of what CAMS can do even in the face of serious suicidality.

A Word about Deliberate Self-Harm Behaviors

I would like to end this discussion of CAMS treatment planning—Section C—with a brief consideration of deliberate self-harm behaviors. As many clinicians have experienced, there are a range of self-harming behaviors in which many patients engage. These behaviors may be indirectly self-harming—for example, my VA patient, who smoked three packs of cigarettes and drank a fifth of vodka per day, routinely driving in excess of 100 miles per hour on the Washington beltway. Other behaviors may be much more directly self-harming, such as an inpatient I worked with whose arms were shredded by severe cutting, leaving large welting scars and permanent damage to her ligaments and tendons. Her chest and legs were also covered with scars of severe self-administered cigarette burns. These notorious behaviors, often referred to as "parasuicidal" behaviors, can prove to be nightmarish to practitioners. Yet, these complex self-injury behaviors—while highly destructive and disfiguring—are not typically intended to end the patient's life. For example, many patients with borderline personality disorder experience highly dissociative states that are rapidly and dramatically remedied by cutting behaviors. In these cases, a person can feel terribly lost and disconnected from reality, the cutting then functionally serves to reconnect the person with reality. Obviously, the "functional" cost of the disfiguring behavior is extremely problematic. Nevertheless, these behaviors can be exceptionally seductive to the suffering patient. But similar to a drug of addiction there is a distinct "high" connected with the behavior as well as psychological habituation and withdrawal. Patients often find they must cut more and deeper to get the same effect and it is hard to quit cutting or burning once one is hooked on the behavior.

While these deliberate self-harm (DSH) behaviors are not suicidal per se, they are obviously problematic and not altogether disconnected from actual suicidal behaviors. Unfortunately, there tends to be a significant degree of overlap between DSH and frank suicidal thinking and behaviors. Sometimes, patients engage in DSH behaviors and get carried away or miscalculate in their self-injury behaviors. Moreover, while borderlines are infamous for frequently engaging in sublethal DSH behaviors, they also can suffer terribly, become acutely suicidal, make attempts, and die by suicide. This overlap can be quite confusing and exceptionally challenging from a clinical perspective.

The CAMS approach was not specifically developed to work effectively with DSH; it has always been my sense that CAMS is better suited to working with issues of frank suicidal ideation and behaviors. But I feel I would be remiss if I did not acknowledge this important clinical concern and address it in some manner. In cases in which the patient's suicidal risk is confounded with various self-harm behaviors it is important to try to assess and treat both the suicidality and the sublethal self-harm behaviors. In this sense it is my recommendation that a separate self-injury treatment strategy be layered into the CAMS treatment plan. In this regard, I would recommend the outstanding treatment approaches developed by Linehan (1993a, 1993b) and more recently by Walsh (2006) who provide excellent and practical ideas pertaining to clinical care and treatment of the DSH behaviors.

COMPLETION OF SSF SECTION D—THE HIPAA PAGE

Section D of the SSF is referred to as the "HIPAA page"—it is the page of the index SSF that includes the main elements of what HIPAA regulations require to maintain an appropriate and complete medical record. To complete the full documentation of the CAMS assessment and treatment plan, this page should be filled in after the index session has occurred.

As discussed in Chapter 2, some of the counseling centers using CAMS and the SSF have chosen to forgo the use of this particular page of the SSF because they work within a developmental—versus psychopathological—model and they indicate to me that they are not required to be HIPAA compliant. I am willing to go along with this perspective, if the key elements of a complete medical record are recorded elsewhere in the patient's file. However, my clear bias is for using the SSF HIPAA form as the complete medical record for Suicide Status patients (i.e., there is no need to replicate similar information elsewhere in the patient's file while they remain of Suicide Status). In other words, for patients on Suicide Status the SSF documentation used in CAMS can serve as *the* medical record. The clinician can then easily convert to routinely used documentation after the patient is off Suicide Status. In my view this is the best approach for creating a very thorough and suicide-specific level of documentation, which invariably helps decrease the potential for malpractice liability. The following brief discussions of the main features of the SSF HIPAA page should further clarify the importance of this particular aspect of Suicide Status documentation in CAMS.

Mental Status Exam

Under HIPAA guidelines there is an expectation that mental health clinicians will routinely assess and document information related to the patient's mental status. Within Section D of the SSF, the evaluation of mental status is made relatively simple such that the clinician needs only to circle certain items and add a few words of explanation. Please note for those not familiar with psychiatry shorthand, "WNL" stands for "within normal limits."

DSM Diagnosis

Even though I have critiqued the overemphasis on diagnosis in relation to suicide risk (Jobes, 2000), I am not antidiagnosis. Diagnoses are crucial for giving clinicians a common language and understanding the treatment possibilities and prognosis. Accordingly, it was important to be able to record a full DSM multiaxial diagnosis on the SSF.

Overall Suicide Risk Level

It is also important from a clinical conceptualization perspective to make an overall professional judgment about the patient's suicidal risk (Maltsberger, 1994). At the end of the assessment day, the clinician must make an informed judgment about the relative risk of suicide and document that clinical formulation in a clear and definitive fashion. This particular five-tiered rating follows from the work of Rudd and colleagues (2001) and an Air Force working group that was dedicated to creating thoughtful recommendations for competent clinical practice with suicidal patients (Oordt, Jobes, et al., 2005).

Case Notes

Finally, the clinician should write a usual case note related to issues of diagnosis, functional status, treatment plan, symptoms, prognosis, and progress to date. This note should be akin to a general progress note that would routinely be entered into a standard medical record (refer to actual case example in Appendix F).

CAMS SUICIDE STATUS

Thus, with the completion of Section D of the SSF the index suicide risk assessment, suicide-specific treatment plan, and medical record documentation within

CAMS is complete. In such a scenario, the suicidal outpatient is now on "Suicide Status." With the CAMS approach, Suicide Status is a method for identifying and conceptualizing the ongoing suicidal risk with implications for ongoing assessments and updates to the treatment plan, which are discussed further in the next chapter.

SUMMARY AND CONCLUSIONS

This chapter has traversed both the philosophy and the concrete clinical procedures of suicide risk assessment and suicide-specific treatment planning within CAMS. I hope the reader has found that CAMS emphasizes a fundamentally different approach to the entire clinical endeavor of assessment and treatment planning in relation to suicidal risk. As noted, CAMS can be used across theoretical orientations and clinical techniques; the approach accommodates the spectrum of treatments that clinicians may use. The CAMS index session sets in motion an ongoing assessment and treatment planning process for the suicidal outpatient. The key to CAMS risk assessment involves the use of the SSF, which is administered side by side with the patient so that we can underscore the importance of a team approach where the clinician, through the eyes of the patient, endeavors to understand the patient's suicidal phenomenology. An additional empirically based risk assessment is also conducted, which then leads into a transitional phase of developing a suicide-specific treatment plan in collaboration with the patient who participates as a coauthor of his or her plan for care (which was amply illustrated by the Air Force case example). As noted, the SSF documentation is crucial to success in CAMS, which is formally concluded by completion of the HIPAA form after the index session. The spirit of CAMS collaboration is fundamentally sparked in the index session, creating a completely different treatment trajectory and launching the birth of a clinical alliance. This alliance is meant to inspire crucial motivation in the patient to ultimately find whole new and better ways to cope with pain and suffering in pursuit of discovering a life worth living.

CHAPTER 6

CAMS Suicide Status Tracking
Assessment and Treatment Plan Updates

Some years ago as director of clinical training of the Catholic University Counseling Center, I was concerned about certain cases that might "fall through the cracks" of our university-based mental health care delivery system. This concern was accentuated by the fact that we had a large number of student clinicians who were relatively inexperienced. Our training program included 10 psychology and social work externship students (typically in their second or third year of graduate school), 6 brand-new second-year Catholic University doctoral students in clinical psychology supervised by psychology faculty in their first clinical practicum, and usually some clinical "associates" who were advanced graduate students seeking additional clinical experience and supervision. Over the course of any academic year it was not unusual to have 16–20 student-level clinicians working in the Catholic University Counseling Center. While all these students-in-training were talented and closely supervised by licensed staff and faculty, we were understandably concerned that a relatively inexperienced clinician might end up handling some very difficult cases. As a suicidologist, I was especially preoccupied with the suicidal cases and felt compelled to find a way to ensure that these particular cases did not fall by the wayside or fly under our clinical supervisory radar.

To this end, the notion of identifying and clinically "tracking" a suicidal case over the course of clinical care became a major focus in our initial SSF research (Jobes et al., 1997) and continued to be emphasized in the course of developing CAMS (Jobes, 1995a, 2000; Jobes & Drozd, 2004; Jobes et al., 2005). As discussed in the last chapter, having collaboratively established the suicidal risk and co-authored a suicide-specific treatment plan in the index session, we have now successfully identified a suicidal outpatient who is considered to be on Suicide Status within the CAMS approach to clinical care. The focus of this chapter centers on Suicide Status, the ongoing session-by-session tracking of the clinical risk and the process of reviewing and potentially revising the treatment plan with the patient. I also address the more concrete procedural considerations of completing the Tracking Forms, Sections A–C, further on in the chapter.

CAMS SUICIDE STATUS: AN OVERVIEW

To pick up where we left off in Chapter 5, a CAMS patient on Suicide Status is understood to be a suicidal patient who has been successfully and collaboratively engaged in his or her own suicide risk assessment and treatment planning in the index session. In other words, the patient and clinician used the SSF to meaningfully assess the patient's suicidal risk, which led to the development of a mutually satisfactory suicide-specific treatment plan that now justifies ongoing outpatient care. Within CAMS, at the end of the index session, patients who are now on Suicide Status are told that the process of assessing and treating their suicidal risk will be ongoing until there is a satisfactory outcome, which means that this intensive focus on suicidality and monitoring of ongoing risk gets appropriately phased out.

The Development of Various Tracking Approaches

The administrative tracking of suicidal risk in the course of working with Suicide Status patients has been done in a variety of ways over the years. I briefly review three major approaches that lead up to what I am now recommending for CAMS.

The Administrative "Tracker" Approach

At the Catholic University Counseling Center we originally had clinicians simply submit a short form to a box in the main office that was monitored on a weekly basis by a graduate student "Tracker." The Tracker monitored all Suicide Status cases and noted progress in a central log book with session-by-session updates as to whether the patient on suicide status (1) had any suicidal *thoughts*, (2) had any suicidal *feelings*, and (3) was *behaviorally* safe (see Jobes et al., 1997). The director of the agency—as well as the researchers—had access to this log book to ascertain at any time during the year how many patients in the agency were on Suicide Status as well as the individual update for each of these patients. This approach worked fairly well, but did involve clinical judgment and a reliance on clinicians to update the Tracker after each session. Not surprisingly, compliance with this approach was variable—some clinicians reliably completed their update slips and put them in the tracking box within minutes of their subsequent sessions, whereas other clinicians had to be hounded each week to update their Suicide Status cases. This often meant that the graduate student Tracker, or me, or both, might have to hunt down the clinician and seek the update directly or leave multiple notes or e-mails trying to prompt a Suicide Status update.

The Case Consultation Meeting Approach

An alternative agency-based model of Suicide Status tracking has been done for some years now with great success at the Johns Hopkins University Counseling Center (Jobes & Flemming, 2004; Peterson, 2003; Rice, 2002; Weinstein, 2002). At Johns Hopkins there is a weekly clinical staff meeting where a particular part of the meeting is dedicated to a review and update of all cases on Suicide Status. This approach is desirable from an agency perspective because the entire staff hears each week from each clinician about all the cases currently being tracked. This process helps staff become familiar with all of the challenging suicidal cases being seen, which proves to be very helpful if a staff member is providing emergency coverage and must deal with one of these cases. Moreover, in the course of reviewing the Suicide Status cases, clinicians who may be struggling with a case can get some quick support and consultation about the management of the case. Again, this approach affords a level of agency-wide monitoring and a log book is maintained, which provides valuable information about the ongoing nature of the case (see Figure 6.1 for a modified copy of what we use at Johns Hopkins University Counseling Center).

For agencies using CAMS center-wide, I think this weekly case consultation approach to Suicide Status monitoring is excellent, particularly if there are some less experienced trainees who are providing some of the care under appropriate supervision. The Catholic University Counseling Center now uses this approach, as do some other agencies using the SSF and CAMS. Historically, the challenge to tracking suicidal cases in a case conference setting was largely "cultural"—the idea that these cases would be openly monitored and discussed by colleagues and peers on a weekly basis was unappealing to some clinicians. When we first introduced the SSF to various clinical settings I often encountered resistance from the clinicians—they complained that the SSF involved too much paper work and tracking gave them a "big brother" sense of being monitored. In more recent years, however, as the use of the SSF and CAMS has become more widely known, the clinicians I train are much more accepting of Suicide Status tracking and the chance to share their work with colleagues. There appears to be an increased

SUICIDE STATUS TRACKING LOG

__Instructions:__ **This log is to be completed following the first session in which a patient reports suicidal thoughts, feelings, or behaviors. (Note: Patients and clinicians must complete the first two pages of the Suicide Status Form during this index session.) This form is to be updated after each successive clinical contact while a patient is on suicide status (please note cancellations and no shows for scheduled appointments). After the second consecutive "risk-free" session (i.e., two consecutive sessions in which the patient has reported no suicidal thoughts, feelings, and behaviors), the clinician should complete the "Suicide Tracking Outcome Form." If the third session is not "risk free," suicide tracking forms are completed until there are three consecutive risk-free sessions.**

Patient: ______________ Patient #: ______________ Clinician: ______________ Supervisor: ______________

Session # (on suicide status)															
Date (write in date)															
Show (S) Cancellation (C) No-Show (NS)	S C NS	S C NS	S C NS	S C NS	S C NS	S C NS	S C NS	S C NS	S C NS	S C NS	S C NS	S C NS	S C NS	S C NS	S C NS
Suicidal thoughts?	Y N	Y N	Y N	Y N	Y N	Y N	Y N	Y N	Y N	Y N	Y N	Y N	Y N	Y N	Y N
Suicidal feelings?	Y N	Y N	Y N	Y N	Y N	Y N	Y N	Y N	Y N	Y N	Y N	Y N	Y N	Y N	Y N
Suicidal behaviors?	Y N	Y N	Y N	Y N	Y N	Y N	Y N	Y N	Y N	Y N	Y N	Y N	Y N	Y N	Y N

Session # / Date	Comments or update:

Suicide Status Tracking discontinued because: ☐ Resolved ☐ Dropped out ☐ Referred out ☐ Hospitalized ☐ Other: ______________

(Write on back for more comments or updates—Use second log form if patient continues beyond 15 sessions.)

FIGURE 6.1. A modified version of the Suicide Status Tracking Log used at Johns Hopkins University Counseling Center.

awareness that this weekly case review can be remarkably supportive and clinically helpful giving the provider a feeling of being less alone with (and stumped by) a difficult case. Furthermore, as liability issues increasingly worry clinicians, there is a clear sense that the level of assessment, ongoing monitoring, and documentation embedded in CAMS could prove to be protective in a malpractice wrongful death scenario.

The Symptom-Based Instrument Approach

As a third example, there is the Air Force outpatient clinic approach, which relied on the routine use of the Outcome Questionnaire–45 (OQ-45) to monitor patients on Suicide Status (Jobes et al., 2005). In this setting, as noted in Chapter 2, an OQ-45 was completed before each clinical contact. Accordingly, the clinician had from session to session updated information regarding overall symptom distress as well as an ongoing index of suicidal ideation—item 8, "I have thoughts of ending my life." I particularly like this approach to suicide tracking because it provides a more consistent and objective index of symptom distress and suicidal risk. Furthermore, a weekly staff meeting can effectively still use such a tool as part of the discussion, such as in the Johns Hopkins model, which involves discussion of the Behavioral Health Measure (BHM) scores each week. The other major virtue of using symptom-based screenings at every clinical contact—beyond useful medical record documentation—is the further potential to use such information for empirical research or quality assurance. For the solo practitioner who may not be working in a larger group, the use of a standardized tool is optimal when tracking a patient on Suicide Status. Again, in CAMS how long a patient is tracked is *always* at the clinician's discretion. But using a standardized measure at every clinical contact that updates useful clinical information related to symptoms and suicidality is very helpful to clinical decision making.

The CAMS Approach to Tracking

As with most developments in CAMS, the recommended approach to tracking of Suicide Status patients has been built on a combination of empirical research, clinical experience, and the input of clinicians (and their patients). Accordingly, what I recommend is the use of a two-page Suicide Tracking Form (see Appendix A, pages 148 and 149). The first page of the form briefly replicates the assessment and treatment planning process conducted in the index session and should be used at every clinical contact for as long as the patient remains on Suicide Status. The second form—the HIPAA page—is similarly used like it was after the index session and should be completed after every Suicide Status session for as long as the patient remains on Suicide Status.

HOW TO USE THE CAMS SUICIDE TRACKING FORMS

Because we have collaboratively assessed the suicidal risk and successfully negotiated the outpatient treatment plan (with a Crisis Response Plan) in the index session, we are now in a position to provide ongoing care in subsequent treatment sessions while the patient is on Suicide Status. This is the where the real work of mental health care begins.

The approach in CAMS is to continue to remain focused on the suicidal risk potential and to direct considerable time and attention to this issue. This is clearly done at the start of each session by a brief assessment of the ongoing risk, and at the end of each session through a thorough review and potential update of the treatment plan. This process is replicated for every clinical contact while the patient remains on Suicide Status. Again, while practices may vary, I strongly encourage the reader to consider using symptom-based screening tools prior to every session as the best means of gathering a quick sense of where the patient is *before* the patient even sits down in session with the clinician.

Section A: Assessment Update

Beyond our continual focus on the problem of suicidality, the clinician must endeavor to attenuate and further develop the spirit of collaboration and joint effort toward shared goals in subsequent sessions. We do this by always greeting patients warmly and welcoming them into the office

Completing the top of the Section A of the Tracking Form is usually very quick—no more than a minute at most. The patient is already familiar with the core SSF Likert rating constructs and there are no qualitative fill-in answers to complete. It is important to emphasize that we want the patient to rate these items in relation to how he or she is feeling *right now*. In the first session after the index CAMS session (and perhaps more), I think it is helpful to again request and use the side-by-side seating arrangement to replicate the experience of the index session. We need to symbolically recreate the relational dynamic—setting the tone—for reengaging the patient. The message is: I remain interested in working closely with you, seeing the world through your eyes. To set up completion of Section A of the Suicide Tracking Form, I typically say:

> "Welcome back, it is good to see you again. As we discussed in our last meeting, we will continue to focus on your thoughts and feelings related to suicide. To do this, I would like for you to complete a very short assessment. At the end of the session, we will also review our treatment plan together. Would it be okay for me to take a seat next to you as I did before? (*handing*

them the assessment sheet on a clipboard) I would like for you to complete the top part, it should only take a minute. These are some of the same items we considered in our last meeting. . . ."

Any spontaneous discussion that may occur while the patient is completing Section A should be encouraged—we want the patient to continue to become familiar with the SSF Likert constructs and to start indexing his or her pain and suffering in relation to these constructs. Because Section A can be completed rather quickly, particularly as the patient becomes more and more familiar with it, the clinician may opt to not use the adjacent seating at the start of the session. But the adjacent seating should always be used at the end of the session when the treatment plan is considered (Section B). Whatever the case, the patient's completion of Section A ratings precedes a normal face-to-face session for most of the remaining hour. The clinician must be sure, however, to transition with at least 10–15 minutes remaining to Section B using the side-by-side adjacent seating arrangement to discuss the ongoing suicidal risk and to review and revise the treatment plan (Section B).

Section B: Evaluation of Suicidal Risk

Thus, at the end of each Suicide Status session, having again requested permission to take adjacent side-by-side seating next to the patient, the clinician should reflect on the content of the session and determine whether the patient continues to have a significant level of suicidal risk and mark the appropriate part of Section B. This process of evaluating the ongoing risk assessment can be done in a relatively transparent manner—it should not be kept from the patient. To that end, the clinician may explain to the patient that the ascertainment of ongoing suicidal risk in CAMS is multidetermined. A session-by-session clinical judgment must be made from various sources of data—obviously the patient's responses to the SSF items, discussion of suicidality during the session, and the between-session behaviors of the patient. This ongoing assessment during suicide status becomes a regular focus of discussion between the patient and clinician. If the situation improves and the ongoing suicidal risk has meaningfully abated, then SSF Tracking Outcome forms would be completed and Suicide Status (and CAMS) would come to an end. Thus, the ongoing assessment of suicidal risk is a very important clinical activity within CAMS that should be made known to the patient. As with other aspects of CAMS, this clinical assessment can be done with a measure of flexibility, adaptations can be made depending on the practitioner's preferences. At the end of each session, however, the clinician's own professional judgment must serve as the definitive assessment bottom line.

I recommend that the ongoing assessment of risk is best done from four sources of data: (1) the self-report rating of suicidal risk on a standardized assessment measure completed immediately prior to the session; (2) the in-session SSF Likert ratings (particularly the behavioral risk of suicide rating); (3) a general consideration of suicidal thoughts, feelings, and behaviors expressed by the patient in session; and (4) the clinician's "gut" sense of the suicidal risk particularly based on the content and process of the session. Let us briefly consider each of these sources of data, which can be readily synthesized into an overall clinical judgment of an ongoing suicidal risk, or alternatively, the clinical resolution of suicidality marking the end of CAMS.

Standardized Assessment

As noted earlier in Chapter 2, I strongly encourage the use of a standardized assessment tool that is completed at each clinical contact before each session. Across these standardized measures, there is a suicide-specific question that typically uses a Likert-type rating scale to assess suicidal ideation. For example, the OQ-45 item 8—"I have thoughts of ending my life"—uses a Likert rating ranging from "never" to "always." For CAMS clinical tracking purposes we are seeking the low-end ratings on these types of scales (e.g., on the OQ we are looking for a 0 or 1 response of "never" or "rarely," respectively). The significance of this approach is twofold—the data are obtained *before* the session and it provides useful documentation for the medical record.

SSF Assessment

The next assessment consideration should be the SSF Likert ratings made at the start of the session. Ideally, we are seeking low ratings for Pain, Stress, Agitation, Hopelessness, Self-Hate, and especially Overall Behavioral Risk of Suicide. If the reader will recall our discussion of the Shneidman Cubic Model of Suicide in Chapter 2 there is an excellent index for judging imminent suicidal risk—defined by maximal ratings of each construct (the 5–5–5 corner cubelet). Therefore, the further the patient's ratings are from 5–5–5, the better (i.e., the lower the risk). As hopelessness is the single best empirically based predictor of completed suicide, lower ratings on this construct are important as well. Our empirical research shows that the Self-Hate construct is more resistant to short-term change, so this particularly rating is less likely to change very quickly in the near term. The overall rating of behavioral risk is the most important of the SSF constructs in determining suicidal resolution. If, for example, a patient is consistently rating a "1," he is communicating directly that he "will not" kill himself—always the clinical and medicolegal bottom line in this business.

Suicidal Thoughts, Feelings, and Behaviors

The assessment process should incorporate in a general sense an evaluation as to whether any suicidal thoughts, feelings, or behaviors continue for the Suicide Status patient. Thus, the clinician must determine the presence of *any* suicidal cognitions—specific active or passive suicidal thoughts of any kind. Suicidal feelings might include a sense of impulsivity, an urgent need to do something self-destructive, or a sense in the patient that he or she deserves to be punished in a self-harming manner. Suicidal behaviors include any self-destructive act that would include attempt behaviors or suicidal "gestures"—any specific behavior preparations for an attempt (e.g., stashing medications) would be considered suicidal behavior. This can generally be done directly or through inference based on discussions within the session itself.

The Clinician's "Gut" Judgment

Although it may not sound very scientific, I think I would be remiss if I did not include what many clinicians routinely use and most often rely on—their "gut" judgment of the risk (see Jobes, Eyman, & Yufit, 1995). In CAMS, with the clear emphasis on collaboration and management of suicidality, we are seeking a sense in the clinician's experience that this patient is truly "on board" the treatment train; fully engaged, motivated, and genuinely trying to find other ways of coping and managing suicidal pain and suffering other than resorting to suicide. This assessment is best formulated over the course of the therapy session based on the content and process of the meeting.

Section B: Tracking Risk to Resolution

As noted, the assessment of the ongoing risk is a crucial activity within CAMS because with *three* consecutive sessions of no suicidality—as determined from the foregoing assessments—triggers the administration of the SSF Suicide Tracking Outcome Forms (see Appendix A). As discussed in more depth in our next chapter, Suicide Status is thus discontinued and CAMS comes to an end. This process is administratively operationalized in the "Patient Status" portion under Section B where the clinician notes whether the suicidal risk has (1) clinically abated, and (2) if so, for how many sessions. The notion of using three consecutive sessions of no suicidality as the criteria for clinical resolution of Suicide Status was first based on research from the psychotherapy research literature, as well as relevant theory and clinical experience (Jobes et al., 1997). Subsequently, the three-session convention was later empirically confirmed with actual cases as a reasonable approach to operationalizing the resolution of a particular suicidal episode (Jobes et al., 2005; Peterson, 2003).

Obviously, using three consecutive sessions as the operational criteria for determining the resolution of suicidality means that there will be a minimum of three sessions beyond the index session for further monitoring of suicidal risk as well as reviewing and revising the treatment plan. It also follows that many cases will take more than three sessions to meet resolution criteria. For example, the average number of sessions to achieve resolution in our Air Force samples was 7.5 sessions with a general range of 4 to 11 sessions for most patients. However, we did have a couple of Suicide Status cases in the Air Force sample, which required 20 to 30 sessions of care before they were both medically separated from the military. Whatever the case, the clinician must assess and indicate on the form the resolution of risk and be sure that it occurs over three consecutive sessions for the case to be considered resolved, thereby triggering the use of the SSF Tracking Outcome forms in the next session (if suicidality is truly remitted in that third session, of course).

Finally, a portion of Section B provides an opportunity to note "Patient Status" in the event of other various possible updates, including (1) Discontinued treatment, (2) No show, (3) Referral to, (4) Hospitalization, (5) Cancelled (appointment), and (6) Other. For any of the preceding situations, the clinician should check the appropriate box and handle the situation as professional practice dictates. For example, if a patient does not show up—particularly a suicidal patient—the clinician should make efforts to contact the patient to schedule a next appointment and document the effort to reconnect with the patient (i.e., a case note can be entered on the HIPAA page, which is discussed later in this chapter). The goal with the Patient Status portion of the Section B is to keep on top of the case and at no time allow the status of the patient to be unaccounted.

Section B: Treatment Plan Review and Revision

Having now thoroughly considered various aspects of CAMS ongoing risk assessment, clinical tracking, and how the resolution of suicidal risk is operationalized, we must now consider the review (and potential revision) of the treatment plan. This process is done collaboratively with the patient at the end of each session for as long as the patient remains on Suicide Status.

On the heels of our discussion with the patient about the ongoing suicidal risk (and the need for further tracking or the potential for resolution), the discussion should naturally turn to a mutual consideration of the treatment plan. As this is an important undertaking, this process will take some time, which is why I recommend carving out 10 to 15 minutes at the end of the session to do justice to the task. This review process serves as a critical check-in with the patient as to how things arc going and whether the Crisis Response Plan (in particular) is adequately managing the patient's suicidal pain and suffering. Thus, the clinician and patient thoughtfully revisit the treatment plan from the previous meeting.

In some cases, it may well be that there is relatively little need for much change in the plan from session to session. Again, similar to the index session, Problem 1 is not negotiable—Self-Harm Potential is still the central concern of CAMS and Outpatient Safety remains the principle goal and objective. The Crisis Response Plan may remain essentially intact if it is working or it can be modified as needed to adapt to the patient's ongoing struggle with suicidality. Similarly, Problems 2 and 3 will likely remain relevant, but these problems, goals, and objectives of the patient's treatment plan can be renegotiated, further modified, and altogether changed as indicated by the patient's progress (or lack thereof). The goal is again to underscore the patient's active involvement in the treatment process; we want the patient to feel that the plan is covered with the patient's fingerprints and that he or she remains coauthor in this enterprise. As was done in the index session, both parties sign their name to the plan before ending the session as a reflection of their shared commitment to the treatment. Similar to the index session, the patient is given a photocopy of the tracking page to take home at the end of each session while on Suicide Status.

Section C: The SSF Tracking HIPAA Page

At each phase of CAMS—the index session, each tracking session of Suicide Status, and at Tracking Outcome—there is a respective HIPAA page that is an important part of the medical record. In terms of Suicide Status tracking, the HIPAA page is filled out after the session to provide the appropriate medical record documentation of the case. This page is virtually identical to the HIPAA page that was completed after the index session, with the same assessments and documentation sections. Again, this documentation can be used as *the* medical record while the patient remains on Suicide Status. The clinician can then use his or her regular documentation once the suicidality is resolved or other case outcomes occur (which we discussed in the next chapter).

SUMMARY AND CONCLUSIONS

The continued focus on suicidality, through session-by-session tracking of the ongoing suicidal risk and review/revision of the suicide-specific treatment plan, is a central pillar of CAMS. By design we mean to keep suicidal risk in the crosshairs of the clinical endeavor, for ourselves and for the patient. This is accomplished by the routine assessment of suicidal risk for patients on Suicide Status at the start of each session and over the course of each treatment session. These sessions are brought to a close by a collaborative reexamination of the patient's treatment plan in case there is need for further refinement or revision. This close attention to suicide risk and the continued emphasis on a suicide-specific treatment are designed to accomplish a central goal—the resolution of suicidal risk via the patient finding alternative ways of problem solving and dealing with pain and suffering. When this goal is achieved, Suicide Status (and CAMS) can be brought to a successful end. Although all cases do not always turn out as we hope, the crucial role of ongoing collaborative assessment, treatment, and tracking offers a compelling means for achieving successful resolution of suicidal risk.

CHAPTER 7

Suicide Status Outcomes
The Completion of CAMS

As noted previously, the CAMS approach to suicidality has a beginning (the index assessment/treating planning session), a middle (a series of Suicide Status sessions of ongoing assessment/treatment plan updates), and an end (the completion of CAMS). It is the outcome of CAMS that we consider in more depth in this chapter as we examine the range of Suicide Status tracking outcomes and how the CAMS approach is brought to a sensible clinical close. As in the preceding chapters, we initially consider the conceptual aspects of clinical outcomes before shifting our attention to the specific procedural aspects of working within CAMS to achieve clinical outcomes.

OVERVIEW TO CLINICAL OUTCOMES IN CAMS

In our clinical research we have consistently seen uniform improvements among Suicide Status patients using the SSF (e.g., Jobes et al., 1997), and in more recent CAMS-specific research (Jobes et al., 2005; Kahn-Greene et al., 2006). This uniform improvement over the course of outpatient clinical care was most evident in relation to reductions in overall symptom distress and in relation to some suicide-specific variables. Current empirical research (Jobes, 2005) is being pursued to better understand the specific mechanisms of CAMS-based therapeutic change—what aspects of the approach make the difference? At this point in our research, we know a few important things about clinical outcomes for suicidal outpatients based on the results of our two most rigorous published clinical studies (Jobes et al., 1997, 2005). For example, we see consistent improvements in overall symptom distress over the course of clinical care across different outcomes; about half of the patients in our studies resolve their suicidal ideation within 6–11 sessions. We know there are variables that can be used to predict certain treatment outcomes, especially positive outcomes (e.g., Fratto et al., 2004; Jobes & Flemming, 2004).

Desirable Clinical Outcomes

When I refer to "desirable" clinical outcomes in relation to CAMS patients, I am referring to optimal suicide-specific treatment-based outcomes that include (1) no completed suicide, (2) no suicide attempts, (3) the elimination of suicidal ideation, (4) the meaningful reduction in general symptom distress, (5) the development of alternative ways of coping, and (6) the development of meaningful reasons for living. Beyond suicidality-related outcomes, we also consider additional clinical outcomes that may occur during care.

Suicidality-Related Outcomes

In terms of clinically preventing suicide completions, suicide attempts, and decreasing suicidal ideation, our existing correlational data can only speak to an apparent relationship between CAMS-based treatment and significant reductions of suicidal ideation over the course of outpatient care (Jobes et al., 2005). The challenges of empirically studying the *causal* impact of any clinical treatment on reducing suicide completions is extremely challenging because of the sample sizes that are required to have sufficient power to detect a statistically low-base rate event such as completed suicide. However, there has been some success from randomized clinical trials research conducted by Linehan (2005) and Brown, Hare, and colleagues (2005) showing that certain cognitive and behavioral treatments can actually reduce the incidence of suicide attempt behaviors over the course of treatment and at follow-up.

To date, however, the best data that we have about CAMS is that it appears to be well suited for decreasing suicidal ideation and potentially doing it more rapidly than standard approaches to care (Jobes et al., 2005). Nevertheless, there is promising additional data on the relationship between SSF/CAMS care and significant pre–post reductions in general symptom distress (Jobes et al., 1997, 2005; Kahn–Greene et al., 2006). Moreover, as noted in Chapter 2, additional correlational data suggest that CAMS treatment is associated with lower health care utilization (i.e., fewer emergency room visits and less primary care appointments). Future research currently under development will be specifically aimed at the potential impact of CAMS-based treatment on improved coping and the enhancement of reasons for living (Jobes, 2005).

What I have seen from data and clinical practice is that CAMS helps many kinds of suicidal patients, but so far it seems that it may be especially well suited for the highest-risk patients—men who may get in fairly agitated depressed states who tend to not reach out to others for help. I can infer from our research and my own clinical experience that these types of patients are competent at killing themselves and appear to be remarkably competent at getting better as well, *if* they are able to seek out appropriate mental health care. This is the same subgroup of suicidal patients to which I have elsewhere referred as acute resolvers (Jobes, 1995a; Jobes et al., 1997). Indeed, in our Air Force sample, we are seeing most of the potential clinical effects of CAMS occurring within a window of 3–11 sessions (mean = 7) in the course of *completely* extinguishing their suicidal ideation. Obviously, we are thrilled with these cases—they make us feel effective, as if we have made a real difference in the patient's life. Moreover, I would at least conceptually argue that this particular group is perhaps at the most significant risk for actually completing suicide (vs. attempting, gesturing, or only ideating). Inversely, however, this line of discussion may mean that CAMS might be less viable for multiple attempters or chronically suicidal ideators—this topic is something we hope to empirically study in the near future.

Continuation of Psychotherapy Post-CAMS

One obvious desirable outcome is the mutual continuation of psychotherapy beyond Suicide Status resolution, which marks the conclusion of CAMS. Over the years I have known many patients who eagerly seek to build on their initial therapeutic success. By conquering their life-and-death struggle, such patients remain highly motivated to continue in psychotherapy. In such cases, the patient and clinician may move seamlessly into an ongoing line of psychotherapy as CAMS comes to a close. While the original work may have been launched by CAMS care, other inherent issues naturally come to the fore as the spotlight on suicidality fades out.

Referral to Other Care

I include making professional referrals as a desirable clinical outcome because I feel so strongly about the importance of skillfully matching patients with the proper clinical care. I spend considerable time referring patients to appropriate care, because I consider making clinical referrals an extremely important professional skill set that is all too often underappreciated as an important part of practice. I also think there are better and worse ways to effect referrals so that the patient does not feel "dumped" but rather feels that he or she has been carefully evaluated, prepared, and transitioned to the best possible care provider. This clinical skill requires particular sensitivity and must be carefully presented in the course of "upstream" discussions that speak to the possibility of a potential "downstream" referral as an indicated and potentially desirable course of action. Thus, a well-made referral is a valuable clinical outcome if it truly means matching the best possible care (and provider) to a well-suited patient who is likely to maximally benefit from that care.

Mutual Termination of Psychotherapy

Another positive outcome is the mutual termination of psychotherapy as CAMS care comes to a close. In our various research studies across samples I would estimate that approximately 20–50% of CAMS patients chose to not pursue additional psychotherapy beyond resolution of suicidality (this was particularly true for our military samples). It has been my experience that for certain patients, a short-term course of care that has a positive outcome and ends on the patient's timetable may be the best way to promote further treatment at a later point in time, if needed. On the other hand, for some patients who have initial CAMS success, there is a clear incentive to continue and build on that success. Either outcome, to continue with psychotherapy or to terminate treatment (without everything being resolved), is a positive outcome if the patient has meaningfully turned a therapeutic corner in the course of a relatively short-term focused line of suicide-specific work.

In my experience, clinicians all too often presume that more psychotherapy is always more desirable. I can think of a number of patients I have seen who self-describe themselves as not being a "therapy-type person." When such a person has short-term success, particularly in a life-and-death struggle with suicidality, I always mention the possibility of termination to ensure that they do not feel "trapped" in endless therapy. In a related sense I usually offer clinical "tune-ups" or "booster" sessions as an alternative option to consider if they are inclined to terminate. I take this approach because experience has taught me that control and autonomy are so often central issues in the suicidal mind, I am therefore particularly sensitive to respecting and honoring those sentiments. Usually, I tend to err on the side of not pushing things further than what we set out to do—in the case of CAMS care, this means having collaborative success in establishing alternative ways to cope with pain and suffering rather than suicide. In my mind, something quite profound has been achieved when we succeed in systematically making suicide functionally obsolete in the life of the patient; that sometimes is enough.

Undesirable Clinical Outcomes

It follows from the foregoing discussion, that there are also a variety of undesirable clinical outcomes that a clinician my see when working with CAMS patients. Without simply rehashing the inverse of desirable outcomes, I would like to highlight a few of the main possible clinical outcomes that are clearly undesirable from a clinical standpoint.

Suicide Completion and Attempts

Of course, we all know that there are no guarantees in this business. It is unlikely that there will ever be a clinical approach or treatment that will always work for every patient and clinician. Having said that, however, I would still strongly contend that a clinical assessment and treatment that specifically targets suicidality is invariably going to do better than a treatment targeting psychopathology where suicidality is understood as a mere symptom. It seems self-evident that a treatment that does not focus on the risk of suicide completions or attempts has a much higher likelihood of simply missing these behaviors. While suicidal behaviors remain a low base rate event, there are always going to be cases where even the most conscientious clinician and approach may not help to avert behaviors that frankly remain largely outside our direct influence and control. If we truly mean to avert suicide, we must keep our eye on the suicidal ball.

Drop-Outs

Among the most worrisome of outcomes are clinical dropouts, which in our studies may account for 15–20% of our samples (e.g., Jobes et al., 1997). Clinical dropouts are a subsample of patients who sought care, acknowledged some degree of suicidal thinking, and subsequently dropped out of that care—not responding to calls, letters, or e-mails encouraging them to return. This situation often leaves the clinician feeling like a failure because a connection was not made with the patient; there was a failure to obviously "hook" the patient to the treatment process. Again, this concern goes to the heart of CAMS philosophy and structure with its clear emphasis on the collaborative involvement of the patient in clinical assessment and treatment planning process—from start to finish.

Hospitalization

As CAMS is expressly designed as an approach to keep suicidal patients *out* of the hospital, it follows that a hospitalization is not a desired outcome event. However, I readily acknowledge that hospitalization is not an undesirable outcome in all cases. On the one hand, I do believe that many—perhaps most—suicidal cases are best handled on an outpatient basis. But I also believe that contemporary clinicians tend to be too oriented toward hospitalization as the optimal clinical response. Nevertheless, if a hospitalization is required to literally save the patient's life, then I think there is no question about its inherent interventive worth. So, this "undesirable" outcome is relative; it is only undesirable when used unnecessarily or prematurely in a case that could have otherwise been better handled on an outpatient basis. By endeavoring to keep patients out of the hospital, we can avert the stigma that is often associated with inpatient care and also create the potential benefit that comes from successfully battling through a rough time without having to resort to the "ultimate" mental health intervention.

Chronic Suicidal States

Based on clinical experience and research, it appears that CAMS maybe less well suited for more chronic suicidal states, particularly in the presence of a borderline personality disorder. Fortunately, there is an effective viable treatment approach for these particularly challenging cases. Over 30 years of empirical research has shown that Marsha Linehan's dialectical behavior therapy (DBT) is the proven treatment of choice for self-destructive borderline patients (Linehan, 1993a, 1993b, 2005; Linehan, Armstrong, Suarez, Allmon, & Heard, 1991). Linehan's work in DBT is impressive and many of her initial findings have now been further replicated by her group as well as others (Linehan, 2005).

Having argued for the primacy of DBT as the best treatment of choice for suicidal borderlines, I would nevertheless anecdotally report that CAMS has shown some value for borderline suicidal patients. There were a handful of cases in our Air Force sample who had personality disorders as well as chronic suicidality (Jobes et al., 2005). In various discussions, clinicians of these patients noted that they felt that even these patients were helped by CAMS. This was because in the course of CAMS care, these particular patients had less of a need to act out or "amplify" their distress through suicidal threats or behaviors because their self-destructive impulses were being so closely monitored by Suicide Status tracking during each and every session. These clinicians insisted that this particular aspect of CAMS was especially helpful in the course of working with these chronic cases even in the face of some very long-term treatments (e.g., 35+ sessions) with little other objective improvement over the course of care.

CAMS SUICIDE TRACKING OUTCOMES: PROCEDURAL CONSIDERATIONS

In terms of specific CAMS procedures related to outcome, there are two primary domains of outcomes to consider: (1) CAMS resolution, and (2) nonresolved clinical outcomes. Each of these domains of clinical outcomes is now considered with a particular emphasis on relevant procedures.

CAMS Resolution

In the previous chapter it was noted that three consecutive sessions of no suicidality—as variously defined by different data sources—triggers the resolution of Suicide Status within CAMS. In those cases in which there have been two such consecutive sessions, the CAMS clinician should be prepared to bring Suicide Status to a close in the subsequent next session, as long as the patient presents as operationally nonsuicidal in that third consecutive session. In the resolution session, the Suicide Tracking Outcome forms (see Appendix A) are administered to formally bring CAMS to an end. To introduce this final phase of CAMS, I typically say:

> "After three consecutive sessions of no-suicidality we are potentially in a position this meeting to bring our Suicide Status tracking to a close as it would appear that suicide as a means of coping with your pain and suffering has been made obsolete by our successful work together. While we will want to be vigilant for the return of any suicidal thinking, I believe we may have turned a significant corner in our work together, which means the completion of a final set of forms and further consideration in this session about where we go from here. . . ."

Having set the stage for resolution, the clinician provides the patient with a copy of the tracking forms for the patient to complete Section A.

Suicide Resolution: Section A

By this time the SSF ratings in Section A are extremely familiar to the patient. While side-by-side seating is always optional, it is probably not necessary in the resolution session. However, there is value in reviewing the SSF items with the patient after the ratings are completed. The clinician may also consider a review with the patient of the SSF index session in order to compare and contrast changes that have occurred over the course of CAMS care. In addition, there is a prompt at the end of Section A for patients to write responses regarding what was helpful about their care as well as what they learned. These two queries have been adapted from those used in the National Institute of Mental Health (NIMH)–funded Collaborative Study of Depression (Elkin et al., 1989) and can be used to generate discussion between the clinician and patient about what has been accomplished.

Suicide Tracking Outcome Form: Section B

When the patient has completed Section A, I take the form back to consider the responses in advance of completing Section B. In relation to evaluating the resolution of suicidality, the key SSF variable to note from Section A is the final (item 6) SSF Likert rating variable of behavioral risk of suicide—*this variable must be rated as a "1" (will not kill self) for resolution to occur.* As noted previously, other data sources may go into the overall clinical judgment of resolution. I personally use a combination of a standardized scale score, the item 6 SSF variable, and my overall professional judgment about clinical progress to date.

If indeed resolution of suicidality has been achieved, I check the appropriate portion under Section B that a third consecutive session of no suicidality has occurred. The clinician should then lead a discussion about the outcome and disposition of the case with the patient. For resolving cases there are four obvious clinical dispositions: (1) continued psychotherapy, (2) mutual termination, (3) the patient's unilateral termination from care, and (4) a professional referral. With each of these potential dispositions, I proceed as I would with any case following my best professional judgment and standard clinical practices. As noted, I am usually fairly supportive of a patient's desire to end care. However, in cases in which my judgment is that termination is not indicated, I clearly share that opinion with the patient but inevitably honor the patient's wish to end treatment unilaterally. If one wanted to be exceptionally thorough in a unilateral case, the mailing of a supportive follow-up letter would have empirical support as an important intervention (see Motto, 1976; Motto & Bostrom, 2001).

Whatever the specific disposition might be, I *always* commend the patient who successfully resolves Suicide Status. I remind them of how it was when we completed the SSF the first time in the index session and how markedly different it is now that they have met criteria for resolution. After 15 years of researching resolution of suicidal states I remain humbled by the magnitude of achieving this significant outcome and I always make that known to the patient in a forthright and complementary manner.

Suicide Tracking Outcome Form: Section C

As per the previous phases of the CAMS process, the outcome phase has its own HIPAA form (Section C). Like the previous two versions for index and tracking respectively, the outcome HIPAA form is virtually identical in content and is completed with obvious reference to the end of CAMS and the transition to the next line of care or other disposition. This is particularly relevant in relation to the documentation transition the clinician will be making because the SSF paperwork will not be used once resolution has been achieved.

Handling the Return of Suicidality

Of course, it is possible for a patient to have a setback after two consecutive nonsuicidal sessions with increased suicidality that may creep back into the clinical picture in what would have been the third consecutive session (which the clinician anticipated triggering clinical resolution). In such cases, the clinician simply does not administer the Outcome Forms, but continues the use of SSF Tracking forms, resetting the resolution clock until the consecutive session resolution criteria are ultimately met. In the case of two consecutive suicidality-free sessions, if there are traces of suicidal ideation in what would have been the third session, the clinician must reset the consecutive session clock with the patient who remains on Suicide Status. In other words, CAMS Suicide Status is only ultimately resolved after a third *consecutive* suicidality-free session.

Alternatively, there may be cases in which a patient successfully proceeds through CAMS care, meets resolution criteria, appropriately completes the Outcome Forms marking the end of CAMS, only to become suicidal once again. This would be considered a new episode of suicidal risk, which prompts the entire process of CAMS being used again from start to finish. In other words, I am not recommending simply going back to Suicide Status tracking but, rather, to treat the recurrence of suicidal risk as a whole new episode where the use of CAMS begins all over again with index session assessment and treatment planning. Not all clinicians may want to start the whole CAMS procedure over from scratch, but I remain convinced that seeing suicidality as episodic is better than simply labeling it "chronic." I believe it is important to impress on the suicidal patient that one can get better (even episodically), which stands in sharp contrast to the perception that things will never be better—the plague of any chronic state.

Unresolved Clinical Outcomes

There are of course many alternative clinical outcomes to resolution or ongoing tracking. As one of the goals of the SSF is to provide a vehicle for documentation that captures the full range of outcomes, the CAMS Tracking Outcome forms may be used for the following outcomes, which are generally linked to a discontinuation of the relationship with the CAMS clinician. These outcomes might include (1) an inpatient hospitalization, (2) a mutual termination between clinician and patient (even without the resolution of CAMS), (3) unilateral termination on the patient's part (dropping out of care or terminating against the wishes of the clinician), and (4) a clinician's referral to other care or a different provider. These outcomes have been discussed throughout the chapter. The clinician is encouraged to seek consultation if needed, form a best professional judgment, make a best professional recommendation for care, and be sure to document well the disposition and specific clinical outcome that results.

SUMMARY AND CONCLUSIONS

This chapter has examined the final portion of the CAMS process—the point at which clinical outcomes are realized and, in the optimal scenario, CAMS is brought to a successful conclusion. There are many alternative clinical outcomes to this optimal scenario that have been reviewed in this chapter. At its best, the resolution of CAMS marks a significant achievement—the systematic deconstruction of suicidality as a means of coping with pain and suffering that leads to the construction of alternative ways of coping. Even when this most desirable of outcomes is not realized, the SSF and CAMS approach can still accommodate the range of possible clinical outcomes, as well as the related documentation therein. Whatever the case, the final phase of CAMS provides an important punctuation mark to the CAMS collaborative process of identifying, engaging, assessing, and managing suicidality. This process reflects an important mutual endeavor between the clinician and suicidal patient to find a compelling alternative to suicide, responding to the patient's needs, and facilitating a kind of healing that may be truly life-saving.

CHAPTER 8

CAMS as a Means
of Decreasing Malpractice Liability

This book has thus far been dedicated to the singular pursuit of life-saving clinical work with suicidal patients. A perhaps unseemly aspect to our efforts is the very real threat of malpractice litigation should we "fail" in our efforts to prevent a patient's suicide. This issue is a major source of contemporary concern for clinicians (at least in the United States). Recent survey data confirm that such concerns are warranted. According to Peterson, Luoma, and Dunne (2002), the majority of family survivors of a loved one in clinical treatment at the time of their suicide death considered contacting an attorney, and 25% actually did. This chapter considers various aspects of malpractice wrongful death tort actions in relation to a patient's suicidal death and we look at how using CAMS with a suicidal patient may address issues of potential negligence, thereby decreasing malpractice liability. Although I know this topic can often dangerously veer toward an overemphasis on protecting ourselves versus the inherent importance of saving lives, we must nevertheless consider the various issues in this chapter because they are so important to competent practice that by its nature *does* help save lives.

OVERVIEW TO MALPRACTICE

It is important to note at the outset of this particular chapter that findings of malpractice liability are based on laws that vary from state to state. In truth, the determination of wrongful death malpractice liability may often be determined by the relative credibility of the engaged experts and the skills of the participating attorneys who influence the sentiments and sympathies of nonexpert jurors. So, while the relevant laws may vary and the relative impact of experts and lawyers cannot be predicted, what is clear in this arena is that responsible and systematic care of patients is very helpful in dissuading attorneys from suing for malpractice in the first place.

As discussed by Berman and colleagues (2006), malpractice wrongful death litigation following a suicidal death is a tort action whereby the plaintiff (usually surviving family members) seeks to pursue malpractice litigation against the clinician-defendant. A plaintiff's complaint is typically filed in civil court usually listing various failures attributed to the clinician-defendant. Within this unpleasant scenario these alleged failures on the part of the clinician—acts of commission or omission—are purported to be either a direct or proximal cause of death or injury.

Whether a clinician is judged guilty of malpractice is determined through the lens of the "standard of care," which is defined as the professional practice that one would expect of a reasonable and prudent clinical practitioner, in similar circumstances, with a similar patient. Notably, the standard of care is *not* what the expert practitioner would be expected to do; rather, it is what the reasonably prudent and generally competent clinical practitioner would do. The situation evolves with court orders to produce all relevant written materials related to the case, a process referred to as discovery. The litigation process then continues with both sides engaging experts who will evaluate the written record to determine whether the clinician did not or did meet the professional standard of care.

From my own experience and from discussions with other forensic experts, the vast majority of these cases do not go to trial. This is largely due to the nature of this type of litigation. It is important to note that plaintiff attorneys spend a great deal of time developing and pursuing a case of malpractice wrongful death that is typically taken on contingency. While plaintiffs pay for costs related to pursuing the case, the lawyer's compensation for their billable hours is contingent on the outcome of the case (i.e., a favorable settlement or a monetary award that arises from a guilty verdict). In other words, the prospect of not recouping billable hours that typically range from $40,000–$50,000 for an average case makes plaintiff attorneys cautious about pursuing just any case (Wise et al., 2005). Thus, many cases initially pursued by grieving families do not progress because plaintiff attorneys are understandably wary of expending significant amounts of time for which they may not be contingently compensated. In the final analysis, while clinician fears and anxieties about malpractice liability are understandable and do have a basis in reality, only a relatively small number of potential malpractice cases ever see the inside of a courtroom (Berman et al., 2006).

The experience of going to court to fight for one's professional life is a dreadful situation. But even if the case does not go to court, the experience of being accused of malpractice will take its toll on the clinician's professional reputation and personal life. As noted by Hendin, Haas, Maltsberger, Szanto, and Rabinowicz (2004), a patient's death by suicide is in itself experienced as a catastrophic event in the life of the clinician, sometimes causing severe distress in the clinician-survivor. Add to that grief the possibility of malpractice litigation and you have a truly miserable experience, making the loss of the patient just that much more unbearable for the clinician.

Having clearly established the aversive nature of the malpractice experience, it is nevertheless instructive to be aware of the actual process and thereby further appreciate what is otherwise expected of clinicians who work with suicidal patients. As noted by Berman and colleagues (2006), for a plaintiff to prove malpractice wrongful death after a suicide has occurred, four central elements must be demonstrated through the litigation process:

1. Evidence must be presented that the mental health clinician had a duty to care (which is typically self-evident through the nature of the professional relationship).
2. Evidence must be presented that there was a dereliction in the clinician's performance of that duty.
3. It must be shown that damages occurred (e.g., various secondary losses such as future income, pain and suffering, and the loss of companionship).
4. Critically, while the specifics vary from state to state, it must be established that these damages were *caused* by the alleged dereliction of the clinician's duty (e.g., through negligence).

Over a decade ago we published a paper that specifically focused on decreasing malpractice liability through competent practice (Jobes & Berman, 1993). It was argued in this paper that competence in relation to the suicidal patient is defined by three overarching principles. These principles of competent professional practice with suicidal patients include the importance of (1) forseeability (assessment), (2) treatment planning (ideally that is suicide-specific), and (3) clinical follow-through (including the importance of consultation and appropriate documentation). This organizing focus for decreasing malpractice liability directly shaped the development of key features of CAMS. Let us therefore generally consider each of these principles in more depth before examining them in relation to CAMS.

THE IMPORTANCE OF FORSEEABILITY

The concept of forseeability pertains to the idea that the clinician anticipated the potential for suicide risk and consequently performed a suicide risk assessment.

However, the thoroughness of the assessment is often a critical issue within malpractice cases. For example, is it *reasonable* for a clinician to ask a 14-year-old with a history of conduct-disordered problems and previous suicidal ideation and behaviors, "are you suicidal" to which the teenager simply responds, "no"? On the one hand, a defendant can legitimately argue, "suicide ideation question, asked and answered." Whereas the plaintiff attorney might effectively argue, "Yes, but can you truly take at face value the answer of this boy given his history?" Frankly, depending on the particular circumstances of each respective case, I have made related arguments on both sides of this debate; it always depends on the specifics of the case as most clearly reflected in the medical record. In reference to the case just mentioned, yes, it is good that the clinician at least asked the 14-year-old about suicide and documented that fact in the medical record. Frankly, many clinicians do not even do this. But will it be enough to convince a judge or jury that the clinician provided an adequate level of "standard care?" This is impossible to answer, as each case has its own unique factors and circumstances. But do you really want to take the risk?

The best strategy for averting the contest of competing forensic expert opinions is simply being sure that you have conducted a very thorough assessment of suicidal risk that is well documented. The CAMS/SSF-driven interview-based assessment of risk is always usefully supplemented by the administration of additional assessment tools. The use of assessment tools and having multiple sources of assessment data are extremely helpful and may be protective from malpractice liability. Obviously, there are criticisms of the demand characteristics of self-report tools; anyone who wants to fake "looking good" can easily do so. As an aside, there may be value in considering the use of other psychological tests that are not as transparent (e.g., the Rorschach) or that have the ability to directly assess the issue of validity in a valid and reliable manner (e.g., the Minnesota Multiphasic Personality Inventory [MMPI]). These assessment measures may or may not directly assess suicide risk, but they can nevertheless be quite revealing about what is really going on with the patient.

Critically, no matter how one chooses to do assessment, there is always value in consistently assessing suicidal risk and making an overall formulation of risk explicit. The suicidal risk should always be well documented on a consistent basis across the full course of clinical care. This overall formulation of suicidal risk should always be explicitly linked to the medicolegal issue of "clear and imminent danger" in particular reference to the need—or not—for hospitalization. Every time the clinician writes a suicide risk formulation, there should always be an explicit discussion of why hospitalization is or is *not* indicated depending on the clinician's judgment, which should always be rooted in the best interests of the patient. Years ago I faced a challenging case of a high-risk suicidal young man who, when he was a teenager, had been repeatedly hospitalized during summers. According to the patient, his parents opted to hospitalize him to go on extended

Caribbean vacations over three consecutive summers. In the course of each of these psychiatric hospitalizations, the patient was brutally and ritualistically sexually abused by two members of the psychiatric nursing staff. Given this traumatic history, I did not believe an additional hospitalization as an adult was in this particular patient's best interest. Fortunately, this patient was successfully treated through some seriously suicidal states by intensive outpatient care. Given the circumstances, my documentation for not hospitalizing this patient was extremely thorough and comprehensive, with extensive discussion of my professional reasoning as to what was truly in the patient's best interest.

Thus, documentation is always crucial. As any plaintiff attorney will tell you: "If it was not written down, it did not happen." Among the clinicians I know and train, the importance of documentation is almost always seen as an onerous and unduly burdensome demand. Yet in a malpractice wrongful death scenario, the lack of documentation can always be turned cruelly against the clinician-defendant by a skilled plaintiff attorney. The plaintiff attorney will point out that explanations about what the clinician did and did not do have no credibility—it is the clinician's word against the suicidal behavior of the deceased patient. An obvious treatment failure. The adversarial tactics, for which plaintiff attorneys are infamous, never put the clinician-defendant in a flattering light. A skillful attorney can easily foment sympathy among the jury for the grieving family in the face of the rich and heartless doctor (whether the clinician is or is not), who was obviously derelict in caring for the patient by virtue of the fact that the patient is now dead. It has been argued that 80–90% of what determines in the mind of the attorney whether a malpractice case should be pursued depends principally on the quality of the written medical record (Wise, Jobes, Simpson, & Berman, 2005). Bottom line, there is nothing more protective than thoughtful competent clinical care that is well documented.

Forseeability and CAMS

Clearly, the idea of identifying suicidal risk at the earliest possible point in the clinical encounter and subsequently assessing that risk thoroughly is a hallmark feature of CAMS. This is particularly true if the clinician is using a standardized symptom-based assessment tool to identify any potential risk through self-report. If current suicidal risk is quickly picked up and identified, thereby triggering the index session use of CAMS, there can be little doubt whether the clinician missed the risk or sufficiently attended to it. In a related sense, it is hard to imagine a practical assessment of suicidal risk that could be more thorough or better documented than the initial use of the SSF with the various quantitative and qualitative assessments of suicidal phenomenology as well as empirically based suicide risk variables.

THE IMPORTANCE OF TREATMENT PLANNING

It is perhaps obvious that the overall formulation of suicidal risk should be used to directly shape the patient's treatment plan. Although this may be obvious, it does not always work this way. From my particular bias, the problem that most concerns me is when a clinician does not sufficiently target the issue of *suicide* in the treatment plan. Again, this may be related to the common practice of seeing suicidality as only a symptom of a major psychiatric illness. While this may be fairly common in practice, it is still problematic because of the seriousness of suicidality. Thus, there is a need to make at least a part of the patient's treatment plan suicide-specific. As I have discussed earlier, a coercive no-suicide contract as it is often used is almost always insufficient to serve as an adequate treatment response or plan for the issue of suicidal risk.

Beyond addressing the issue of suicidality in the treatment plan, the plan should also identify both short- and long-term treatment goals. In the cases in which suicidality exists, there must be a short-term strategy to manage outpatient stability and safety as well as a strategy for what the patient should do if a crisis state arises. Articulating the short-term contingencies of the treatment is always valuable. Beyond this more immediate press for short-term contingencies and stability, the treatment plan should also address longer-term overarching goals as well. Although it is likely that short-term treatment goals are more important overall, being mindful of the longer-term treatment goals—the clinical big picture—demonstrates both a balanced and a thoughtful approach to treatment planning.

A common complaint that is often seen in malpractice litigation is failure on the part of the clinician to recommend appropriate and necessary treatments. This is the "Monday-morning quarterbacking" by the plaintiff's expert, who with the clarity of hindsight knows all the things that *should* have been done to save the deceased. For example, not referring a patient with significant symptoms of a mental illness for a psychiatric medication consultation could be viewed as a major act of clinical omission. Following this particular example, even if a clinician does not believe in the worth of psychotropic medications—and makes that argument citing relevant research—the clinician may nevertheless be found liable for malpractice. The current position of most forensic experts would be that referrals for medication consultation reflect the professional standard of care. Therefore, the failure to make such a referral could have liability implications— whether the patient takes the referral or not is another matter altogether.

Beyond the issue of treatment omissions, the clinician's consideration and referrals to the full spectrum of treatments generally demonstrate a broader and more comprehensive approach to clinical care. In hindsight, such an approach appears more protective in contrast to a narrower approach that exclusively relies on only one treatment (particularly when there is evidence that an additional referral or an alternative treatment *could* have made a difference). For example, with suicidal adolescents the failure to have substance abuse separately evaluated by a specialist might be argued in hindsight by the plaintiff's expert as a significant failure. This would be particularly true if substance abuse was an obvious significant contributor to the suicidal risk. All these considerations emphasize the core value of making all clinical decisions in relation to the patient's best interest, but additional consideration should be given to potential worst-case scenarios. I am convinced that it is possible to always practice in the patient's best interest first and foremost while still being mindful of liability and what can realistically be done to decrease the clinician's potential liability in a worst-case scenario. What I know to be true from my workshops is that many clinicians are "scared" into seeking additional training in clinical suicidology primarily because of their fear of malpractice litigation. But if the net result is that this fear compels a clinician to adopt a broader and more comprehensive approach to care, then liability concerns have served to improve practice, which should always be good news for the patient.

It is also very important to revise and update a patient's treatment when indicated. Sometimes when a case is going poorly there is a need to completely overhaul the entire treatment plan. This discussion goes to the importance of staying on top of the treatment and not settling into an open-ended treatment where the retrospective review of the forensic expert will render an opinion that the treatment plan was outdated, inadequate, and not appropriately modified to the evolving clinical realities and needs of the patient. Clinicians who can demonstrate that their treatment was dynamic, creative, and evolving in the face of clinical demands—and as reflected in the documentation of the case—are much less vulnerable to malpractice liability.

Beyond the constant refrain about the importance of documentation there is a need to routinely seek professional consultation on difficult cases (which of course should always be carefully documented). The importance of professional consultation cannot be overstated. Professional consultation is critical because it demonstrates good clinical judgment and the appropriate use of one's resources and makes clear that the clinician was not operating as a "lone ranger" on the case.

A final general consideration alluded to earlier is the potential importance of seeking a release from the patient to obtain collateral information and support from family members and possibly other important people in the patient's life. For example within our military research we often observed the significant positive impact of engaging the patient's first sergeant or commanding officer in an effort to problem-solve job-related problems or interpersonal issues within the patient's unit (as we saw earlier in the case example depicted in Chapters 4 and

5). Alternatively, engaging parents and siblings of a suicidal teen can be crucial in creating a supportive safety network around the patient. Spouses can be similarly engaged to great effect. Although there are exceptions where engaging significant others is not a good idea, one should routinely consider the virtue of pursuing collateral information/support as a standard part of clinical care.

Treatment Planning and CAMS

Clinical treatment planning that is relevant to suicide risk is not an issue in CAMS because the CAMS treatment plan is principally about the potential risk of suicide. While other issues are addressed in the course of working with patients on Suicide Status, work on other concerns is virtually always in service to the main goal of CAMS, which is to fundamentally eliminate self-harm behavior as a means of coping with pain and suffering. Moreover, the treatment plan in CAMS is never static. For as long as the patient remains on Suicide Status, the CAMS treatment plan is explicitly reviewed and updated as needed at *every* single clinical contact.

THE IMPORTANCE OF CLINICAL FOLLOW-THROUGH

A final concept of competent practice—with implications for decreasing malpractice liability—pertains to the importance of clinical follow-through. Thus, competent clinical treatment, which should always be reflected in the written record, requires the clinician to execute the treatment as planned and to professionally follow through, working on behalf of the patient. An obvious and important forensic question is the determination of whether the treatment that was planned was actually implemented. I have seen several forensic cases in which the treatment plan that appeared in the medical record reflected an appropriate and adequate approach to the case, but the clinical care that actually ensued did not comply with the plan. Such a treatment plan follow-through failure may be directly linked to the patient's demise and tends to confirm liability on the part of the clinician.

Another major complaint that is routinely seen in malpractice cases is a failure to coordinate care with other providers involved in the patient's care. A corollary to this is that one should always at least attempt to make contact with the patient's previous care providers. Of course, these contacts must always be documented. Most commonly in this particular arena is a breakdown that often occurs between a psychotherapist and a physician who is prescribing and monitoring the patient's medications. Naturally all appropriate releases, signed by the patient, authorizing this coordination of care should be in the medical record as well. In addition, provisions for emergency coverage should be noted. Documentation about clinical coverage and mindfulness about potential emergencies reflects professional awareness, conscientiousness, and clinical competence.

When effecting a referral to another mental health professional, one should always be careful to develop the rationale and timetable leading up to that referral. Obviously the ethical issue of clinical abandonment must be carefully considered and managed. This concern is particularly true in cases in which the patient is reluctant to accept a referral from the clinician. If the clinician's judgment is that this referral is in the best interest of the patient, then the rationale for the referral must be developed and documented in the medical record. Any follow-up documentation that describes the outcome of the referral (e.g., whether the patient accepted the referral) is important information to include in the medical record.

It is my understanding that in some jurisdictions, there may be provisions in state laws that make it possible to maintain notes that are separate from the medical record progress notes, which are required and may be discoverable. It is therefore important to be aware of jurisdictional statutes as to whether under HIPAA provisions and state law the clinician is allowed to maintain a separate set of nondiscoverable psychotherapy (or process) notes. If the clinician is allowed to maintain such notes, they should do so because these notes typically provide a much more detailed level of practice that can be produced to verify the depth and thoroughness of care, which may not be typically reflected in medical record progress notes. However, the clinician must be sure to follow the relevant rules or statutes that pertain to maintaining personal notes. For example, such notes must typically be stored in a completely separate file (i.e., these notes must be physically stored in a different location away from the patient's medical record). These kinds of personal or process-oriented notes tend to be more narrative in nature and can accommodate a much more detailed level of content and information than the typical progress notes of the medical record, which tend to highlight just the facts of the case.

Follow-Through and CAMS

Another hallmark feature of CAMS is clinical follow-through. In fact, the CAMS approach is all about follow-through. The issue of suicide should never "fall through the cracks" of clinical care for Suicide Status patients managed by CAMS. The ongoing clinical tracking of suicidal risk is a constant focus, for both the clinician and the patient, over the entire course of CAMS care. The SSF is basically a follow-through roadmap. If the clinician faithfully completes each section of the SSF at the beginning, through the middle, and at the end of CAMS he or she has been compelled to routinely assess suicidal risk, attend to a suicide-specific treatment plan, consider the use of referrals, and seek professional consultation. Use of the SSF means that the clinician is HIPAA compliant and by using CAMS the clinician has produced a remarkably complete and thorough suicide-specific medical record, *par excellance*. More important, however—which is the whole point of this undertaking—the clinician will have provided outstanding clinical care to the suicidal patient.

SUMMARY AND CONCLUSIONS

As noted through this chapter, competent practice, working in the patient's best interest, and being mindful of potential malpractice liability are not mutually exclusive concepts. If a clinician works to thoroughly assess suicide risk, thoughtfully develop a treatment plan specific to that risk, and follow through on clinical care, the clinician will have provided a level of quality care that far eclipses the "standard of care"—the lens that is used to examine malpractice liability. If the clinician uses CAMS there will be competent clinical practice that is abundantly documented and suicide-specific. CAMS lays out a clinical course of action before the clinician and patient for them to collaboratively pursue together. It is my deep sense that this kind of practice will make a difference in the life of the struggling patient by fundamentally helping to preserve that precious life, which is the best possible protection from wrongful death malpractice liability.

CHAPTER 9

Future Developments

Using CAMS across Settings and Future Research

In this final chapter I consider a variety of possible future developments related to CAMS both in terms of its application across various settings and in relation to empirical research. As noted early on, the development of the SSF and its ultimate use within CAMS arose out of real-world clinical needs. For the most part this need was originally inspired among outpatient psychotherapists working in university counseling centers with suicidal students and later among Air Force mental health providers working with active-duty personnel in outpatient clinics. Ultimately, direct clinical needs in conjunction with ongoing empirical research shaped the development of CAMS. In other words, there was never any grand *a priori* vision about developing CAMS; it arose out of necessity and was shaped by clinical and empirical data. CAMS as it now exists will continue to evolve particularly in relation to its use in additional mental health settings and in relation to evolving research.

THE USE OF CAMS ACROSS CLINICAL SETTINGS

CAMS is intended to be flexible and adaptable to a wide range of clinical settings. As noted throughout the book, CAMS tends to heavily emphasize a focus on suicide risk assessment that cuts across a range of settings. Beyond risk assessment,

CAMS is further designed to accommodate a broad range of treatments for suicidal patients. What follows is a discussion of a few such settings in which CAMS may be effectively imported and used.

Hotlines and Crisis Centers

I have considered the possible use of the SSF and the CAMS approach to suicidality within crisis center and hotline work (e.g., Jobes, 2004a). Obviously, some adaptations are needed to use CAMS in crisis center settings. For example, on a telephone hotline the crisis counselor will not literally be taking a seat next to the caller to complete the SSF because they are sitting on two ends of a phone line. Nevertheless, the potential use of the SSF as a guide for the hotline worker's assessment of suicidal risk is a natural application of these materials. Moreover, even without being physically in the same space, the overarching philosophy of the CAMS approach can still be effectively applied to a suicidal caller. In my experience many paraprofessional hotline counselors have excellent suicide-specific assessment and counseling skills, sometimes even better than some mental health professionals who often do not receive suicide-specific training in the course of their graduate, medical, or nursing training (Bongar, 2002). Hotline workers know well that they must have suicide-specific training, because they encounter the issue so frequently in their work.

Over the years I have been approached by many crisis center directors who are interested in using the SSF, as well as applying CAMS to their settings. Anecdotally, I know that the ideas represented in this book have been used with great success in crisis center work. But to date, there has neither been any systematic adoption of SSF/CAMS in crisis centers nor any empirical research of its use in these settings. However, given recent research by Mishara and colleagues (2005), there are a number of compelling reasons to consider using these materials (e.g., as a means of systematically structuring and standardizing paraprofessional assessments and interventions with suicidal callers).

Outpatient Clinics

Because the SSF was originally conceived—and CAMS was later developed—in outpatient mental health clinics, their uses are naturally well suited to these clinical settings. As previously noted, CAMS is particularly valuable in situations in which there might be concerns about suicidal patients "falling through the cracks." For example, in settings in which less experienced clinicians may be engaged in supervised training, use of CAMS provides valuable structure and support. Moreover, the routine use of Suicide Status tracking—particularly in conjunction with a staff case conference review—requires clinicians to stay on top of these cases. I know in the settings in which we have implemented the SSF and CAMS, the agency directors feel significantly reassured that worrisome suicidal cases are being appropriately identified, managed, and accounted for. Moreover, the use of an agency log book enables a director or any staff member to have specific knowledge of all the suicidal cases being seen at any point in time.

Colleagues in Denmark have successfully used CAMS in an outpatient mental health clinic setting that is linked with the Copenhagen County University Hospital. A recent 2-year grant was obtained to develop and clinically implement CAMS to 30 suicidal outpatients using a Danish translation of the SSF. My Danish collaborators have been quite enthused about their use of CAMS in this outpatient setting. There are some potentially interesting cross-cultural differences in Danish SSF qualitative responses and we are further studying perspectives gained from their use of CAMS within this clinic.

Community Mental Health Centers

Over the years I have provided training and consultation to a number of community mental health centers (CMHCs). Through my interactions with these professionals I have gained a sense of the unique needs and challenges of these settings and I believe there is real potential for using CAMS in community mental health. One problem raised by a number of community mental health professionals is that the SSF and CAMS may be too sophisticated for work with the severely mentally ill or the cognitively disabled patients. Although this is an understandable concern, I would contend that clinicians can use the SSF as a valuable clinical guide even with more severely disabled patients. However, for CAMS to be used successfully with more disturbed patients, it will likely require more time and a very active and directive level of involvement by the clinician. In my own practice I have successfully used CAMS with delusional and psychotic patients—but it has required more patience, time, and perseverance on my part. For cognitively disabled patients, or for those who do not read, the clinician can still use the approach, but again the clinician must simply be much more active in terms of walking the patient through each element of the SSF. I understand that many clinicians do not have the luxury of time that is required to administer the SSF and CAMS to such patients. This may be particularly true for clinicians in CMHC settings who may have inordinately large case loads of sometimes very sick patients. Another issue shared by some CMHC clinicians (above and beyond impossibly large and complex caseloads) is that they often find themselves swamped in copious amounts of administrative paperwork. At this point it should be quite clear that using CAMS involves a great deal of documentation, which may simply overwhelm the CMHC clinician who already feels unduly awash in paperwork.

Private Practice Settings

It is my belief that CAMS—and this book—may be particularly well suited to private practice clinical settings. I know from my workshop training experiences, that private practitioners often report feeling particularly vulnerable to working with suicidal patients. Depending on the nature and scope of the practice, the private practice clinician may feel uniquely isolated as many private practitioners often do not have a staff of colleagues or administrative support staff that creates structure and a valuable sense of professional support. Many private practitioners describe feeling at a loss with a new suicidal patient or when an existing patient becomes suicidal, which means they often find themselves trying to figure things out as they go. Even with good intentions and a genuine desire to help, these practitioners sometimes get in over their head, not knowing how to proceed with a suicidal case, which can increase the potential for "suicidal blackmail" (discussed in Chapter 3).

As a compelling alternative, CAMS can directly and efficiently help the private practitioner by providing a clear procedural roadmap, a means for maintaining appropriate documentation, and a clinically useful framework for successfully proceeding with a suicidal patient. I routinely receive dozens of calls and e-mails each year from private practitioners I have trained who attest that using CAMS has singularly transformed their practice life in relation to working with suicidal patients.

Forensic Settings

To date the SSF has been used minimally in forensic settings. Over the years I have provided training and consultation to mental health providers at a maximum-security prison in Maryland. Clinical work in such a setting is a very different undertaking—working with a convicted felon who faces a 30-year prison term creates some inherently challenging problems for the clinician. To be sure, issues related to suicide risk are particularly complex in forensic settings. On the one hand, incarceration—whether it be a lockup, jail, or prison—objectively increases the statistical risk of completed suicide considerably (Maris, Berman, & Silverman, 2000). On the other hand, the threat of suicide can be instrumentally used as a means of getting oneself out of the general cell block population and into the relative "comfort" of the prison medical ward. Accordingly, clinicians in these settings struggle mightily with discerning genuine versus manipulative (instrumental) suicidal risk. Add to this mix the politics of mental health care in forensic settings and the issues of liability should a patient die by suicide and we find ourselves working in one of the most challenging settings imaginable.

My sense is that CAMS could be effectively used in such settings for three principle reasons: (1) there are typically no time pressures; usually clinicians can work open-endedly with these patients as long as there is some progress; (2) the thorough assessment of risk using the SSF in CAMS may be helpful in discerning genuine versus feigned suicidal risk; and (3) CAMS documentation may prove to be particularly helpful from a liability standpoint.

Emergency Departments

The issue of time is particularly pressing in emergency departments where a doctor may have only 10 minutes to evaluate a patient. Nevertheless, my colleague in Switzerland who uses CAMS to assess ER patients in a Zurich hospital reports that it takes him about 10 minutes more to use the SSF in a side-by-side CAMS-oriented assessment. But he insists that what he loses in time, he gains in the cooperation and engagement of the patient. I am currently only aware of ER use of Sections A and B of the SSF for successfully assessing acute suicidal risk. Data collection is now under way to assess the effectiveness of using this portion of the SSF in ER settings versus more traditional approaches. Anecdotally, this adaptation of CAMS to the emergency room seems to be promising.

Current research is also being pursued with colleagues at the University of Washington to use CAMS to increase compliance with "next-day appointments" (NDAs). For ER cases of suicide attempters or acutely suicidal patients in which inpatient hospitalization is not indicated, the use of an NDA is a potentially compelling option for patients who do not have a mental health care provider. The problem is, however, that the majority of patients who are given post-ER NDAs do not attend the scheduled appointment. It is our sense that using an index CAMS-based interview in the ER to set up the NDA will markedly improve the likelihood that patients will attend follow-up appointments, thereby improving treatment engagement and compliance with improved clinical outcomes overall (Comtois, Jobes, & Morgan, 2005).

Employee Assistance Programs

There are two employee assistance programs (EAPs) that have used the SSF in recent years. Given the fundamentally short-term nature of EAP work, the index use of the SSF and CAMS-based suicide-specific treatment planning is very well suited to EAP work. Given that EAP clinicians usually only have one to four sessions with an employee-client, the initial use of CAMS is very useful but Suicide Status tracking and resolution is probably less applicable. As before, the rigorous CAMS documentation is always valuable.

Inpatient Settings

There are currently two inpatient settings in which the SSF and CAMS are being used with considerable success. At the Mayo Clinic in Rochester, Minnesota, nursing staff has reliably administered the SSF upon admission, which has meaningfully shaped patients' treatment plans (Lineberry et al., 2006). I had the unique experience of a first-year resident at Mayo excitedly recounting using the RFL and RFD assessment from the SSF to completely refocus the treatment on a patient's particular psychosocial stressors. For the patient—and his doctor—it was nothing less than a clinical epiphany.

Similarly in Switzerland, we are seeing success in using CAMS with inpatient samples. As described by Schilling, Harbauer, Andreae, and Haas (2006), 45 suicidal inpatients were given a German translation of the SSF using the CAMS approach. These authors noted impressive decreases in overall symptom distress and suicidal risk over the course of inpatient stays that typically lasted about 10 days. However, according to within-subjects analyses, apparent pre–post clinical improvements were markedly weaker among patients with a previous history of suicidality and high levels of posttraumatic stress. While this kind of within-subjects research is limited in the absence of comparison control groups, I am nevertheless pleased to see the apparently successful development and implementation of CAMS in real-world clinical settings (particularly across different cultures). Of course in future research we hope to be able to randomly assign patients to CAMS and alternative clinical conditions to compare both treatment process and outcomes.

FUTURE DEVELOPMENTS AND EMPIRICAL RESEARCH

Our research over the past few years demonstrates that CAMS can and will continue to evolve for many years to come as we continue to learn more and more about clinically working with suicidal states using the SSF and CAMS approach. This chapter ends with a brief review of future developments and where our research is heading in the coming years.

Technology

A major area for future development relates to technological advances that should make using CAMS with a suicidal patient easier and more efficient. The most obvious technological development would pertain to using an electronic version of the SSF either on a laptop or using an electronic notepad. We are currently working with experts to develop an electronic SSF that could export both quantitative and qualitative data into a patient's electronic medical record. Obviously Suicide Status tracking can be greatly facilitated and made more reliable with the use of pop-up windows that prompt the clinician to administer the proper SSF form creating a comprehensive electronic medical record. A striking development in recent years with the Veterans Affairs medical health care system has been extraordinary advances in the area of electronic records—a true model of technological health care innovation that has created direct benefits for patient care. It is inevitable that electronic versions of assessment and medical record-keeping will become the norm and I anticipate that CAMS will fit well into that level of innovation.

In a related vein, it is also inevitable that as we continue our treatment-oriented CAMS research, we will probably one day have algorithms that can be used to predict potential treatment outcomes for patients engaged in CAMS. To some extent we have already done certain early versions of this type of research (Fratto, Jobes, Pentiuc, Rice, & Tendick, 2004; Jobes et al., 1997; Jobes & Flemming, 2004; Peterson, 2003). One recent unpublished study shows the potential for using microanalytic intensive designs along with sophisticated data analyses (Kahn-Greene et al., 2006). In this study we empirically investigated trajectories of treatment improvement for a sample of 92 suicidal college student outpatients who were treated at the Counseling Center at Johns Hopkins University in Baltimore, Maryland. In this agency where CAMS is routinely used, patients are also required to complete BHMs at every session. By using hierarchical linear modeling we were able to determine whether index SSF ratings (e.g., the six Likert scales) could be used to determine if any particular construct moderated eventual treatment effects. As shown in Figure 9.1, we see differential reductions in the frequency of suicidal thoughts (depicted on the y axis) over the course of outpatient treatment sessions (depicted on the x axis). The figure shows the statistical probability of decreases in suicidal thoughts that is differentially determined by the sixth SSF rating scale of overall risk of suicide. More specifically, when patients in this sample rated the SSF overall risk relatively high (e.g., a "3" or a "4" on the 5-point Likert scale), it took more sessions to reduce suicidal thoughts (up to 17 sessions). In contrast, those patients who gave relatively lower SSF overall risk ratings had more rapid reductions in suicidal thinking (in the 5–8 range of sessions). Interestingly, this differential effect was significantly moderated by SSF ratings of hopelessness and self-hate.

Future research with much larger samples of suicidal outpatients will enable us to combine all the SSF assessment constructs—both quantitative and qualitative from Sections A and B—into linear treatment model analyses to determine what index variables might tell us about the unique suicidal risk of any one

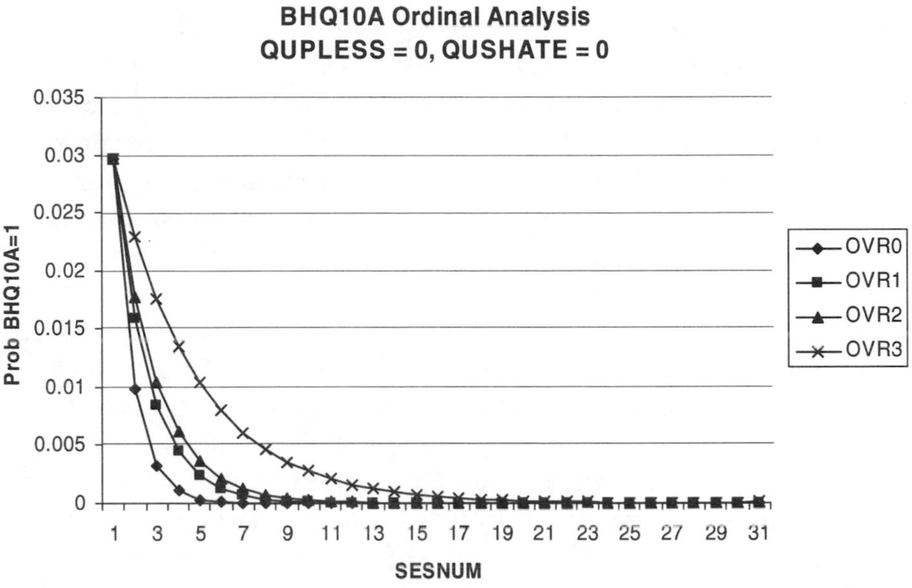

BHQ10A Ordinal Analysis
QUPLESS = 0, QUSHATE = 0

FIGURE 9.1. The relationship between index SSF ratings of overall risk of suicide (the sixth SSF rating scale) on differential reductions in suicidal thoughts over the course of psychotherapy sessions.

patient, and ultimately what particular aspects of treatment should be emphasized for the best outcomes.

Someday it will be possible to collaboratively complete an electronic version of the index SSF with a suicidal patient and promptly run the results through research-based software. The output of this analysis would indicate certain possible outcomes and guide possible aspects of treatment by providing a menu of treatment options particularly well suited to the patient's idiosyncratic suicidal state. Such software could provide an empirically informed version of electronic consultation. This kind of technological evolution of CAMS offers an incredibly exciting prospect for clinicians and patients alike.

Assessment Research

Our existing data suggest compelling research opportunities to further advance our ability to assess suicidality. Overall, we plan to pursue more information about the inherent nature of suicidal risk and suicidal typologies. For example, we have established across a number of studies a suicidal patient profile of a good candidate for rapidly resolving suicidal ideation (Fratto et al., 2005; Jobes et al., 1997; Mann, 2002; Peterson, 2003; Rice, 2002). What we have determined at this point is that the rapid responder is (1) someone in acute distress with an intense need for escape, (2) less likely to have a previous mental health history, (3) less likely to write much on our qualitative SSF assessments, (4) more likely to be a male who is psychologically "entrapped" (Williams, 2001), (5) markedly constricted in their thinking, and (6) otherwise a potentially competent person who is not currently problem solving very well. Across our studies such patients reliably respond quickly to outpatient care, resolving their suicidal ideation and decreasing overall symptom distress (Jobes et al., 1997, 2005; Kahn-Greene et al., 2006).

An interesting twist to the preceding data was seen in yet another counseling center study where we simply counted the number of words used to respond to the various SSF qualitative prompts (Jobes & Flemming, 2004; Peterson, 2003). In other words, given the finite opportunity to respond to the SSF Likert scales, the RFL versus RFD, and the One-Thing response, we could see if "expansive" responders (those who wrote a lot) had a different outcome from "constricted" responders (who wrote very little). In this study we saw a wide-ranging word count from 0 to 226 words with a mean of 75 words per SSF. Interestingly, and unexpectedly, we found that chronically suicidal and hospitalized patients had significantly high word counts in comparison to those who resolved their suicidal ideation in short order (or dropped out). We anticipate doing a great deal more of this type of qualitative research because it may speak to distinct differential treatment outcomes related to a kind of "psychological immersion" in suicidality versus those more constricted responders who appear to not have as much to say about their suicidal suffering.

Additional or more specific suicidal subtypes have been more difficult to identify through our existing assessment research. For example, overall we have been less successful in our efforts to understand more fully various subgroups with the less desirable results (e.g., the particularly worrisome treatment dropouts). Thus a goal in our future assessment research will be to develop empirically based profiles that better identify for the clinician possible concerns. For example, if a patient shares a profile with a typical dropout, extra effort could be extended to thoroughly engage and "hook" that patient to care. Moreover, we are beginning to see data that help us deconstruct various aspects of suicidal states—for example, some data suggest meaningful differences between dysphoric versus agitated suicidal people, which may indicate neurobiological differences needing different psychosocial and medication treatments (Jobes & Bostwick, 2006).

Treatment Research

The preceding discussion of using assessment data to reliably identify suicidal subtypes opens the door for empirically developing treatments that uniquely address the idiosyncratic needs of certain suicidal states. Both research and practice demonstrate that different mental health conditions require different treatments. Through future research we hope to develop a menu of empirically based treatment approaches that will specifically treat certain types of suicidal risk.

CAMS Clinical Trial Research

Currently a primary focus for CAMS-related research is the pursuit of clinical trial research. To date, our existing data have been retrospective and correlational. Although the preliminary data have been encouraging (Jobes et al., 2005; Kahn-Greene et al., 2006), we are still not in a position to empirically say that CAMS *causes* a reduction in suicidal ideation or behaviors. To be able to talk about a causal effect on suicidality requires the gold standard of clinical treatment research—the randomized clinical trial (RCT) design. As previously noted early on in this book, RCTs for the treatment of suicide are remarkably few. For example, Linehan (2005) notes that with 35 RCTs published in the professional literature on treating suicide there are almost as many published RCTs for spider phobics! In 20 years of practice, I have never seen a spider phobic, whereas I have seen many suicidal people. The challenges of doing prospective treatment research on suicide are considerable. Add potential liability to the critical concern of losing a person to suicide and it is understandable why so many researchers have avoided this topic. Yet, we must pursue more empirical work in this area if we ever hope to make a difference—something that Linehan has been strongly advocating for some years now.

In my own pursuit of RCT research on CAMS, I have learned a number of important lessons that relate to conducting this challenging research and bear directly on the current text. In recent efforts to pursue grant funding to study CAMS in an RCT, it became clear that the version of CAMS that had been developed to date could not be used in a fundable prospective RCT. By design the existing version of CAMS was meant to be flexible and *not* be seen as a free-standing treatment for suicidality. The goal to date has been to *not* dictate treatment to clinicians so that CAMS could be used widely across theoretical disciplines. Thus CAMS as a clinical assessment and engagement framework remains unique and valuable for all the reasons I have been listing since page 1. But this flexible and eclectic approach to CAMS does not meet the necessary criteria to be able to formally call the approach a "treatment" (that could then be studied in a prospective RCT). Therefore, the process of writing a grant proposal in part led directly to the present book, which emphasizes the eclectic use of CAMS. Throughout the book, I have emphasized our research to date on the SSF and early development of the CAMS approach and have taken great pains never to say that CAMS is a *treatment*. To legitimately call CAMS a treatment, prospective RCT research is needed, which in turn requires the development of a whole new CAMS-based treatment (that can be largely built on the ideas and empirical work represented in this book).

CAMS Problem-Solving Treatment

Currently under development is "CAMS Problem-Solving Treatment" (CAMS-PST)—a proposed 12-session stand-alone *treatment* for suicidal ideation and behaviors. Our goal is to develop and study the potential effects of CAMS-PST on samples of suicidal outpatients within prospective RCT research designs. As proposed thus far, CAMS-PST begins with the ideas embodied in this book but adds a specific emphasis on problem solving related to suicidogenic issues. In other words, building on our qualitative SSF Likert research, CAMS-PST clinicians will focus on those issues that our data indicate are central to the suicidal patients we have studied (Jobes et al., 2004). For example, as discussed in Chapter 2, we know that patients in our studies have suicidal issues related to relationships, vocational issues, issues of self, and emotional struggles. As per the proposed CAMS-PST manual, clinicians will emphasize a focus on these four areas of concern. The CAMS-PST process of care would emphasize the central dynamic of collaboration that would be applied to the following five domains over the course of 12 sessions:

1. Collaborative SSF Assessment
2. Collaborative SSF Treatment Planning
3. Collaborative Deconstruction of Suicidogenic Problems
4. Collaborative Problem-Solving Interventions
5. Collaborative Development of Reasons for Living

If we are able to further develop and study CAMS-PST using RCT methodologies there will undoubtedly be many advances in the continuing evolution of CAMS. At this juncture, however, work on CAMS is proceeding on two tracks that are meant to address different needs and achieve different goals. With the first generation of CAMS described in this book there is an assessment-focused clinical framework that clinicians can now use to better manage suicidal patients, accommodating a range of possible treatment approaches. In contrast, the next generation of CAMS—CAMS-PST—may be able to provide a structured but flexible problem-solving approach for clinicians who are seeking an empirically developed and effective treatment (obviously, only if our future clinical trial research confirms this to be true).

Training Research

Finally, one additional exciting frontier in clinical suicidology is work and empirical investigation in the area of professional training. As an active professional trainer, I have been involved in significant system-wide training efforts in the Air Force (Oordt, Fonseca, Schmidt, & Jobes, 2005) and more recently in the Veterans Affairs health care system. We have data from the Air Force that demonstrates that we can create pre–post training differences in knowledge and attitude toward working with suicidal patients, including changes in clinician behaviors at 6 months of follow-up (Oordt et al., 2005). I have long been involved in training efforts through the AAS, which in recent years is bringing a thoughtful focus to professional training as a major area of emphasis. Critically, the use of research will greatly help us shape and target our training efforts so that we may discern what information, in what modality, is best imparted to make the biggest difference in clinical reality.

SUMMARY AND CONCLUSIONS

These are exciting days for working with CAMS in relation to new developments, applications/uses in different settings, innovation, and future empirical research. Sixteen years of steady research on the SSF and now CAMS has begun to yield useful data that has been described at length in this book. I know there is material in this book and within this approach that will make a meaningful difference to readers and to their patients. But the biggest potential breakthrough on the horizon is linked to future RCT investigations that may be able to demonstrate that beyond assessing, tracking, and managing suicidal states, an evolved version of CAMS may be shown to decrease suicidal ideation and behavior in a causal manner. Given the seriousness of suicidality and challenges inherent in treating it, achieving that particular goal would undoubtedly be worthwhile. I truly believe that through collaboration all things are possible, not the least of which is coaxing a life to be meaningfully lived back from the jaws of a suicidal death. I believe this singular pursuit is both a noble and crucial undertaking if we are ever to clinically conquer the scourge of suicide in the patients we see in practice.

Epilogue

The term *asylum* was originally based on the French word *asile* meaning a place of refuge (Goldstein, 1993). It was Jean-Etienne-Dominique Esquirol who originally coined the term when he proposed the formation of new institutions in France that would be specifically used for housing the insane. Mentally ill people who roamed the streets and alleys of medieval European cities were routinely rounded up and thrown in jails, restrained in dark cellars, and mixed with various deviants. Early 16th-century efforts to "care" for the mentally ill in the asylums of France, Spain, and Portugal were not exactly humane (Millon, 2004). Indeed, some asylums early on were open to the public for viewing mentally ill people as if they were animals in a zoo. Suicidal people in this era (and for years to come) were treated cruelly. During medieval times, for example, the body of a person who died by suicide was often dragged into the street, left to decay, or pinned down with a stake through the heart to keep the soul from rising and possessing other persons.

Over the centuries, however, a bit more compassion was extended to the suicidal "lunatic." Such people were increasingly seen as victims of suicidogenic influences of society. In turn, more enlightened notions of care evolved over time. Theoretically, asylums came to be conceptualized as protective environments where vulnerable suicidal patients could be kept safe and given sanctuary. In due course asylums evolved into mental hospitals as medical and treatment-oriented approaches began to take root in the 19th and 20th centuries.

In the late 1800s Sigmund Freud began making his mark by inventing the "talking cure" and diverse forms of psychological talk therapies developed over the ensuing century to the present day, providing a range of approaches for working with mental illness and suicidality. When Thorazine was first introduced in the 1950s to manage psychotic symptomatology, an indisputable mental health revolution was born. The explosion of psychoactive medications that were developed over the next 40+ years had an immeasurable impact on how mental illness was conceptualized, assessed, treated, and clinically managed with momentous and far-reaching implications for providers and patients. Many of these developments gave mental health professionals a growing sense of confidence that mental illnesses could be helped through appropriate diagnosis and treatment. Yet specific treatments for suicidal risk lagged and the automatic use of hospitalization, often with lengthy stays, was the intervention of choice for virtually any patient who whispered the presence of suicidal thoughts.

In the latter portion of the 20th century, relatively routine and established clinical practices within mental health care began changing dramatically. The idealistic community mental health movement of the 1960s preceded a period of rapid deinstitutionalization of state mental hospitals during the 1980s, which of course was followed by dramatic changes ushered in by managed care in the 1990s. In the course of recent changes, the basic clinical wisdom that suicidal people *belong* in hospitals has not corresponded to realities brought on by deinstitutionalization and managed mental health care. As a result of these changes, hospitalizing patients has become too expensive—we can no longer afford to protect people from themselves as we once did. Furthermore, thousands of mentally ill people who would have lived in institutions only decades ago now find themselves living in the street or incarcerated in jails and prisons—not unlike their predecessors of the Middle Ages. While we would like to think that we are highly evolved in how we care for the mentally ill and suicidal, in some ways, we have come full circle right back where we started. Too many suicidal people continue to suffer and too often receive limited or inadequate care, which sometimes results in death by suicide.

We clearly know that the clinical challenges inherent in working with suicidal states are considerable. Limitations on our ability to hospitalize suicidal patients have greatly narrowed our options. The ever looming threat of malpractice in the wake of a suicide terrifies many clinicians. We are indeed navigating through some difficult and treacherous waters these days when it comes to clinically encountering a suicidal person. Yet one must have a reasonable response; we can neither avoid suicidal cases nor simply give up.

The CAMS approach described in the book is thus designed to provide one such reasonable response. The approach is designed to be a thoughtful and measured way for dealing with these contemporary challenges. In CAMS we work to recognize the legitimate need of the suicidal person to escape unbearable suffering. Our empirical data confirm what the enlightened Europeans theorized—that suicidal patients do need refuge; they need psychological asylum, a sanctuary from the torments of their struggle. CAMS is thus designed to help provide that needed refuge by fostering a therapeutic collaboration between the clinician and suicidal patient that engenders a form of psychological asylum in the form of a strong *outpatient* clinical relationship. This collaborative relationship is meant to inspire motivation in the patient for finding new and better ways of coping, such that the life that originally seemed utterly unlivable may come to be seen as potentially viable. By using CAMS, the clinician and patient can endeavor to create the patient's life anew—a life enriched by meaningful relationships, work, and a sense of self in the world.

Finally, at the end of the therapeutic day, it is not enough to just survive in life; that is no way to live. On the other hand, survival is an important start. But for our suicidal patients to truly make it in the land of the living, they must go beyond mere survival to finding *their* way to live and perhaps even one day to *thrive*. I believe this noble goal can be realized through a true collaborative therapeutic effort that enables the suicidal patient to choose life even in the face of daunting psychological pain and suffering. This joint therapeutic effort—the backbone of the CAMS approach—enables the team to work together to unearth the roots of suffering so that new seedlings of potential hope and a truly livable life can be sown, nurtured, and grown into therapeutic fruition.

Suicide Status Form–III (SSF-III)

*Assessment, Treatment Planning, Tracking,
and Outcome Forms*

SUICIDE STATUS FORM–III (SSF III) INITIAL SESSION

Patient: _____ Clinician: _____ Date: _____ Time: _____

Section A (*Patient*):

Rate and fill out each item according to how you feel <u>right now</u>.

Rank Then rank items in order of importance 1 to 5 (1 = most important to 5 = least important).

_____	1) **RATE PSYCHOLOGICAL PAIN** (*hurt, anguish, or misery in your mind; **not** stress; **not** physical pain*): Low Pain: 1 2 3 4 5 :High Pain What I find most painful is: _____
_____	2) **RATE STRESS** (*your general feeling of being pressured or overwhelmed*): Low Stress: 1 2 3 4 5 :High Stress What I find most stressful is: _____
_____	3) **RATE AGITATION** (*emotional urgency; feeling that you need to take action; **not** irritation; **not** annoyance*): Low Agitation: 1 2 3 4 5 :High Agitation I most need to take action when: _____
_____	4) **RATE HOPELESSNESS** (*your expectation that things will not get better no matter what you do*): Low Hopelessness: 1 2 3 4 5 :High Hopelessness I am most hopeless about: _____
_____	5) **RATE SELF-HATE** (*your general feeling of disliking yourself; having no self esteem; having no self-respect*): Low Self-Hate: 1 2 3 4 5 :High Self-Hate What I hate most about myself is: _____
N/A	6) **RATE OVERALL RISK OF SUICIDE:** Extremely Low Risk: 1 2 3 4 5 :Extremely High Risk (will <u>not</u> kill self) (will kill self)

1) How much is being suicidal related to thoughts and feelings about <u>yourself</u>?   **Not at all: 1 2 3 4 5 :completely**

2) How much is being suicidal related to thoughts and feelings about <u>others</u>?   **Not at all: 1 2 3 4 5 :completely**

Please list your reasons for wanting to live and your reasons for wanting to die. Then rank in order of importance 1 to 5.

Rank	REASONS FOR LIVING	Rank	REASONS FOR DYING

I wish to live to the following extent: Not at all: 0   1   2   3   4   5   6   7   8 :Very much

I wish to die to the following extent: Not at all: 0   1   2   3   4   5   6   7   8 :Very much

The one thing that would help me no longer feel suicidal would be: _____

Section B (*Clinician*):

Y N Suicide Plan:
When: _____ _____
Where: _____
How: _____ Y N Access to means
How: _____ Y N Access to means

Y N Suicide Preparation   Describe: _____

Y N Suicide Rehearsal   Describe: _____

Y N History of Suicidality

  • Ideation   Describe: _____

    • Frequency   _____ per day   _____ per week   _____ per month

    • Duration   _____ seconds   _____ minutes   _____ hours

    • Single Attempt   Describe: _____

    • Multiple Attempts   Describe: _____

Y N Current Intent   Describe: _____

Y N Impulsivity   Describe: _____

Y N Substance Abuse   Describe: _____

Y N Significant Loss   Describe: _____

Y N Interpersonal Isolation   Describe: _____

Y N Relationship Problems   Describe: _____

Y N Health Problems   Describe: _____

Y N Physical Pain   Describe: _____

Y N Legal Problems   Describe: _____

Y N Shame   Describe: _____

Section C (*Clinician*): OUTPATIENT TREATMENT PLAN (Refer to Sections A & B)

Problem #	Problem Description	Goals and Objectives Evidence for Attainment	Interventions (Type and Frequency)	Estimated # Sessions
1	*Self-Harm Potential*	*Outpatient Safety*	**Crisis Response Plan:**	
2				
3				

YES _____ NO _____ Patient understands and commits to outpatient treatment plan?

YES _____ NO _____ Clear and imminent danger of suicide?

_____   _____   _____   _____
Patient Signature   Date   Clinician Signature   Date

MENTAL STATUS EXAM (circle appropriate items):

ALERTNESS: ALERT DROWSY LETHARGIC STUPOROUS
OTHER _____

ORIENTED TO: PERSON PLACE TIME REASON FOR EVALUATION

MOOD: EUTHYMIC ELEVATED DYSPHORIC AGITATED ANGRY

AFFECT: FLAT BLUNTED CONSTRICTED APPROPRIATE LABILE

THOUGHT CONTINUITY: CLEAR & COHERENT GOAL-DIRECTED TANGENTIAL CIRCUMSTANTIAL
OTHER: _____

THOUGHT CONTENT: WNL OBSESSIONS DELUSIONS IDEAS OF REFERENCE BIZARRENESS MORBIDITY
OTHER: _____

ABSTRACTION: WNL NOTABLY CONCRFTF
OTHER: _____

SPEECH: WNL RAPID SLOW SLURRED IMPOVERISHED INCOHERENT
OTHER: _____

MEMORY: GROSSLY INTACT
OTHER: _____

REALITY TESTING: WNL OTHER: _____

NOTABLE BEHAVIORAL OBSERVATIONS: _____

PRELIMINARY DSM-IV-R MULTIAXIAL DIAGNOSES:

Axis I _____

Axis II _____

Axis III _____

Axis IV _____

Axis V _____

PATIENT'S OVERALL SUICIDE RISK LEVEL (check one and explain):

☐ No Significant Risk   Explanation: _____
☐ Mild
☐ Moderate   _____
☐ Severe
☐ Extreme   _____

CASE NOTES (diagnosis, functional status, treatment plan, symptoms, prognosis, and progress to date):

_____

_____

_____

Next Appointment Scheduled: _____   Treatment Modality: _____

_____   _____
Clinician Signature   Date   Supervisor Signature   Date

SSF-III SUICIDE TRACKING FORM

Patient: _____ Clinician: _____ Date: _____ Time: _____

Section A (*Patient*):

Rate each item according to how you feel right now.

1) **RATE PSYCHOLOGICAL PAIN** (*hurt, anguish, or misery in your mind; **not** stress; **not** physical pain*):
Low Pain: 1   2   3   4   5   :High Pain

2) **RATE STRESS** (*your general feeling of being pressured or overwhelmed*):
Low Stress: 1   2   3   4   5   :High Stress

3) **RATE AGITATION** (*emotional urgency; feeling that you need to take action; **not** irritation; **not** annoyance*):
Low Agitation: 1   2   3   4   5   :High Agitation

4) **RATE HOPELESSNESS** (*your expectation that things will not get better no matter what you do*):
Low Hopelessness: 1   2   3   4   5   :High Hopelessness

5) **RATE SELF-HATE** (*your general feeling of disliking yourself; having no self-esteem; having no self-respect*):
Low Self-Hate: 1   2   3   4   5   :High Self-Hate

6) **RATE OVERALL RISK OF SUICIDE:**
Extremely Low Risk: 1   2   3   4   5   :Extremely High Risk **(will _not_ kill self)   (will kill self)**

Section B (*Clinician*):   Resolution of suicidality: ☐ 1st session   ☐ 2nd session
Complete SSF-III Suicide Tracking Outcome Form after third <u>consecutive</u> resolved session

Y ___ N ___ Suicidal Thoughts?

Y ___ N ___ Suicidal Feelings?

Y ___ N ___ Suicidal Behaviors?

<u>Patient Status:</u>
☐ Discontinued treatment ☐ No show   ☐ Referral to: _____
☐ Hospitalization   ☐ Cancelled ☐ Other: _____

TREATMENT PLAN UPDATE

Problem #	Problem Description	Goals and Objectives Evidence for Attainment	Interventions (Type and Frequency)	Estimated # Sessions
1	*Self-Harm Potential*	*Outpatient Safety*	**Crisis Response Plan:**	
2				
3				

_____   _____   _____   _____
Patient Signature   Date   Clinician Signature   Date

Section C (Clinician Postsession Evaluation):

MENTAL STATUS EXAM (circle appropriate items):

ALERTNESS: ALERT   DROWSY   LETHARGIC   STUPOROUS
OTHER: _____

ORIENTED TO: PERSON   PLACE   TIME   REASON FOR EVALUATION

MOOD: EUTHYMIC   ELEVATED   DYSPHORIC   AGITATED   ANGRY

AFFECT: FLAT   BLUNTED   CONSTRICTED   APPROPRIATE   LABILE

THOUGHT CONTINUITY: CLEAR & COHERENT   GOAL-DIRECTED   TANGENTIAL   CIRCUMSTANTIAL
OTHER: _____

THOUGHT CONTENT: WNL   OBSESSIONS   DELUSIONS   IDEAS OF REFERENCE   BIZARRENESS   MORBIDITY
OTHER: _____

ABSTRACTION: WNL   NOTABLY CONCRETE
OTHER: _____

SPEECH: WNL   RAPID   SLOW   SLURRED   IMPOVERISHED   INCOHERENT
OTHER: _____

MEMORY: GROSSLY INTACT
OTHER: _____

REALITY TESTING: WNL OTHER: _____

NOTABLE BEHAVIORAL OBSERVATIONS: _____

DSM-IV-R MULTIAXIAL DIAGNOSES:

Axis I _____

Axis II _____

Axis III _____

Axis IV _____

Axis V _____

PATIENT'S OVERALL SUICIDE RISK LEVEL (check one and explain):

☐ No Significant Risk   Explanation: _____
☐ Mild
☐ Moderate   _____
☐ Severe
☐ Extreme   _____

CASE NOTES (diagnosis, functional status, treatment plan, symptoms, prognosis, and progress to date):

_____

_____

_____

Next Appointment Scheduled: _____   Treatment Modality: _____

_____   _____
Clinician Signature   Date   Supervisor Signature   Date

SSF-III SUICIDE TRACKING OUTCOME FORM

Patient: _____ Clinician: _____ Date: _____ Time: _____

Section A (*Patient*):

Rate each item according to how you feel <u>right now</u>.

1) **RATE PSYCHOLOGICAL PAIN** (*hurt, anguish, or misery in your mind;* **not** *stress;* **not** *physical pain*):   **Low Pain:**   **1 2 3 4 5**   **:High Pain**
2) **RATE STRESS** (*your general feeling of being pressured or overwhelmed*):   **Low Stress:**   **1 2 3 4 5**   **:High Stress**
3) **RATE AGITATION** (*emotional urgency; feeling that you need to take action;* **not** *irritation;* **not** *annoyance*):   **Low Agitation:**   **1 2 3 4 5**   **:High Agitation**
4) **RATE HOPELESSNESS** (*your expectation that things will not get better no matter what you do*):   **Low Hopelessness:**   **1 2 3 4 5**   **:High Hopelessness**
5) **RATE SELF-HATE** (*your general feeling of disliking yourself; having no self-esteem; having no self-respect*):   **Low Self-Hate:**   **1 2 3 4 5**   **:High Self-Hate**

6) **RATE OVERALL RISK OF SUICIDE:**
            Extremely Low Risk: **1 2 3 4 5**   **:Extremely High Risk**
            (will <u>not</u> kill self)   **(will kill self)**

Were there any aspects of your treatment that were particularly helpful to you? If so, please describe these. Be as specific as possible.

_____

_____

_____

What have you learned from your clinical care that could help you if you became suicidal in the future?

_____

_____

_____

Section B (*Clinician*):

Third consecutive session of resolved suicidality: Yes _____ No _____ (if No, continue Suicide Status Tracking)

<u>**OUTCOME/DISPOSITION**</u> (Check all that apply):

_____ Continuing outpatient psychotherapy _____ Inpatient hospitalization

_____ Mutual termination _____ Patient chooses to discontinued treatment (unilaterally)

_____ Referral to: _____

_____ Other. Describe: _____

Next Appointment Scheduled (if applicable): _____

_____   _____

Patient Signature   Date   Clinician Signature   Date

Section C (*Clinician Outcome Evaluation*)

MENTAL STATUS EXAM (circle appropriate items):

ALERTNESS: ALERT   DROWSY   LETHARGIC   STUPOROUS
OTHER: _____

ORIENTED TO: PERSON   PLACE   TIME   REASON FOR EVALUATION

MOOD: EUTHYMIC   ELEVATED   DYSPHORIC   AGITATED   ANGRY

AFFECT: FLAT   BLUNTED   CONSTRICTED   APPROPRIATE   LABILE

THOUGHT CONTINUITY: CLEAR & COHERENT   GOAL-DIRECTED   TANGENTIAL   CIRCUMSTANTIAL
OTHER: _____

THOUGHT CONTENT: WNL   OBSESSIONS   DELUSIONS   IDEAS OF REFERENCE   BIZARRENESS   MORBIDITY
OTHER: _____

ABSTRACTION: WNL   NOTABLY CONCRETE
OTHER: _____

SPEECH: WNL   RAPID   SLOW   SLURRED   IMPOVERISHED   INCOHERENT
OTHER: _____

MEMORY: GROSSLY INTACT
OTHER: _____

REALITY TESTING: WNL   OTHER: _____

NOTABLE BEHAVIORAL OBSERVATIONS: _____

DSM-IV-R MULTIAXIAL DIAGNOSES:

Axis I _____

Axis II _____

Axis III _____

Axis IV _____

Axis V _____

PATIENT'S OVERALL SUICIDE RISK LEVEL (check one and explain):

☐ No Significant Risk   Explanation: _____
☐ Mild
☐ Moderate   _____
☐ Severe   _____
☐ Extreme   _____

CASE NOTES (diagnosis, functional status, treatment plan, symptoms, prognosis, and progress to date):

_____

_____

_____

Next Appointment Scheduled: _____   Treatment Modality: _____

_____   _____
Clinician Signature   Date   Supervisor Signature   Date

Coding Manual for the SSF Likert Scales

Qualitative Assessment

CODING MANUAL:
A CATEGORIZATION OF SSF QUALITATIVE VARIABLES—PAIN, STRESS, AGITATION, HOPELESSNESS, AND SELF-HATE

OVERVIEW

This coding manual will serve as a guide for examining open-ended, qualitative responses provided by suicidal outpatients on an assessment instrument called the Suicide Status Form (SSF; Jobes et al., 1997). The SSF is a suicide risk assessment instrument used at several local university counseling centers. It consists of six self-report and clinician-report items that measure a client's suicide risk. Specifically, the SSF includes ratings of five valid, reliable, and theoretically based items (on 5-point, low-to-high Likert scales) thought to underlie suicidal behavior (Jobes et al., 1997). These include: Psychological Pain, Stress, Agitation, Hopelessness, and Self-Hate. In addition, a sixth item examines a patient's overall behavioral suicide risk. The client is also given the opportunity to provide written open-ended responses that explain the five constructs. The following coding procedure specifically focuses on these qualitative responses and provides a way to categorize client's responses to the five stem cues following each of the Likert items.

GENERAL GUIDELINES FOR CODING

Coders will receive five separate stacks of responses on index cards. These five stacks will represent each of the coding constructs: Pain, Stress, Agitation, Hopelessness, and Self-Hate. First, coders will go through an initial sort of the cards for each construct (one construct at a time) placing responses under the appropriate coding category. After this initial sort of each of the five main constructs, a second sort will be allowed so that coders can review their initial coding decisions and revise them as needed before making their final coding choices. In order for researchers to understand the decision-making process, we ask that coders discuss their rationale for coding decisions.

The categories within each construct should be considered mutually exclusive of one another. Therefore, each response should be placed in *one* category. While some interpretation may be required when deciding on the best category for a given response, generally, coders should take the response "at face value" without giving too much thought into the motivations or situation that may surround the response.

For each response, coders are also asked to rate their confidence in the code they have assigned. A confidence rating of 1 indicates a low confidence level, 2 indicates a medium confidence level, and 3 indicates a high confidence level.

SPECIFIC GUIDELINES FOR CODING

We ask that you please feel free to use the manual as needed because certain decision rules specific to each category are included in the manual.

If two types of responses are mentioned in a single response, place it in the category of the *first* response identified. For example, if the response says "my job and my depression" then place the first response, "my job" in its proper category, but if the response reads, "my depression and my job" then place "my depression" in its proper category.

Please note that some of the constructs may have one or more categories in common. It is important however, that each construct's category is reviewed carefully, as ones that may be very similar in definition may also have critical nuances specific to that item that will affect coding decisions. For example, more than one construct has a "Future" category; however, these definitions are not the same, so please be mindful of critical differences that may affect your decisions.

WHAT ARE THE CODINGS USED FOR?

Coding the five SSF variables will enable those involved in this line of research to identify common categories into which these responses might fall. Theoretical, research, and clinical implications of these qualitative data can guide researchers and clinicians to more accurately assess a person's suicidal risk as well as possibly tailor a client's treatment to address his or her idiosyncratic experiences and needs.

PAIN (PSYCHACHE)

The Psychological Pain variable in the SSF (Jobes et al., 1997) is based on Shneidman's (1993) construct of "psychache." Shneidman purports that the most basic ingredient of suicide is psychache. Psychache is intrinsically psychological and it refers to the hurt, anguish, soreness, aching, and psychological pain of the mind. Psychache is a necessary force in leading a person into a suicidal crisis. Suicide occurs when the psychache is deemed intolerable or unbearable to a person, so suicide is a combined movement toward cessation and a movement away from this intolerable emotion. More specifically, this psychological pain arises out of the frustration of one's vital psychological needs (e.g., affiliation, nurturance, and understanding), whereas these vital needs are ones whose frustration cannot be tolerated. Suicide then can become a direct means of ending one's pain.

There is a somewhat elusive and ill-defined quality of psychache (Shneidman, 1993). Attempts to describe psychological pain have resulted in definitions of intolerable emotions (Murray, 1938); aloneness (Adler & Buie, 1979; Maltsberger, 1988); anxiety, self-contempt, and rage (Maltsberger, 1988); and a more global distress (Derogatis & Savitz, 1999). These may be important contributors to psychache, but Shneidman (1993) argues that they do not capture the inherent complexity and multidetermined nature of psychache. Therefore, the stem phrase **"What I find most painful is. . ."** was added to the Psychological Pain item on the SSF to further elucidate to both patients and clinicians the true phenomenology and the idiosyncratic quality of a suicidal person's psychological pain.

Coding Categories (Total of 7)

1. Self

This category refers to responses that are specific to one's self, or when a reference to one's self is clearly inferred. These can be statements about feelings or qualities about the self. These tend to include descriptions of enduring traits, core attributes, or harsh self-critiques or external descriptors about the self.

> **Examples**:
> "I am such a loser."
> "I can't do anything right."
> "Being overweight."

2. Relational

This category refers to responses that make references to specific relationship problems or issues with children, spouse, partner, parents, friends, significant others, or any other social interaction. Any response that speaks to being hurt by others or hurting others goes here; specific references about being alone or isolated also go here.

> **Examples:**
> "My family is so messed up."
> "Loneliness."
> "Having no friends."

3. Role/Responsibilities

This category refers to responsibilities or obligations related to common adult role expectations including the role of the worker, homemaker, or student. Responses may be specific examples of a role or responsibility or may be an expression of feeling inefficient in these roles. Responses such as academic concerns, financial burdens, or job concerns are included here. Specific future-oriented statements regarding career are also included. Statements that refer to lack of direction or purpose should be placed in the Helpless category.

Examples:
"Have no idea what kind of job I want to get after school."
"I can't decide on a job."
"I suck at being a parent."
"My house is a mess."

4. Global/General

This category refers to nonspecific, broad statements that are completely inclusive and therefore vague. These responses indicate a general, all-encompassing, or overarching sense of being overwhelmed and/or unable to cope.

Examples:
"Seems like everything."
"Life in general."
"The world is a total pain."

5. Helpless

This category refers to implied or specific references to feeling out of control, trapped, or lost. References to feeling directionless are also in included in this category. General statements about hopelessness about one's inability to cope, function, or achieve in the future should be placed here.

Examples:
"I am so out of control."
"I feel so trapped."
"I will fail no matter how hard I try."

6. Unpleasant Internal States

This category refers to specific, discrete descriptions of hurting, distress, suffering, emotional pain, and other negative emotions in the mood spectrum. They are symptom-oriented responses, and are more state-like than trait-like. These responses are free of intrasubjective self-references (e.g., "I hate myself because I always worry.") and are not global (e.g., "Everything makes me sad.").

Examples:
"Depression."
"My nervousness."
"This misery."

7. Unsure/Unable to Articulate

This category refers to responses in which the person is uncertain or unable to respond. It may include responses that seem purposely evasive, avoidant, or apathetic.

> **Examples:**
> "Don't know."
> "Not sure."
> "Who cares?"

STRESS (PRESS)

The Stress variable in the SSF (Jobes et al., 1997) is based on Shneidman's (1993) construct of "press," which was developed from Murray's (1938) work on the theory of press. Press refers to those aspects of the inner and outer world or environment that move, touch, impinge upon, and significantly psychologically affect an individual. Stress or press can then be a facilitating force driving some individuals toward a suicidal crisis, particularly when one experiences multiple sources of stress repeated over long periods of time. Presses can be either positive or negative and include what are termed *beta presses*—an individual's perception of a specific aspect of the environment—or *alpha presses*—the objective or real aspects of the environment. Presses can facilitate or impede the efforts of an individual to reach a given goal; in other words, the press of an object is thought of in terms of what it can do *to* or *for* the person. By understanding presses, we can know more about what a person may do if we have a picture of his or her motives or directional tendencies combined with a sense of the way in which he or she views or interprets the environment. Thus, the stem phrase **"What I find most stressful is . . ."** was added to the Stress item on the SSF to identify and describe suicidal patient's self-reports about the most meaningfully descriptive categories of stresses.

Coding Categories (Total of 8)

1. Relational

This category refers to responses that make references to specific relationship problems or issues with children, spouse, partner, parents, friends, significant others, or any other social interaction. Any response that speaks to being hurt by others or hurting others goes here; specific references about being alone or isolated also go here.

> **Examples:**
> "Making my family proud about my new job."
> "My girlfriend is pulling away from me."
> "I don't have any friends here and I feel like an outsider."

2. Self

This category refers to responses that are specific to one's self, or when a reference to one's self is clearly inferred. These can be statements about feelings or qualities about the self. These tend to include descriptions of enduring traits, core attributes, or harsh self-critiques or external descriptors about the self.

> **Examples:**
> "I'm not a good person."
> "I am unable to lose 10 pounds."
> "I'm weak and too emotional."

3. Role/Responsibilities

This category refers to responsibilities or obligations related to common adult role expectations including the roles of the worker, homemaker, or student. Responses may be specific examples of a role or responsibility or may be an expression of feeling inefficient in these roles. Responses such as academic concerns, financial burdens, or job concerns are included here. Specific future-oriented statements regarding career are also included. Statements that refer to lack of direction or purpose should be placed in the Helpless category.

Examples:
"Having no idea what kind of job I want to get after school."
"I can't deal with thinking about my future."
"I can't handle being at home all day with the kids."

4. Unpleasant Internal States

This category refers to specific, discrete descriptions of hurting, distress, suffering, emotional pain, and other negative emotions in the mood spectrum. They are symptom-oriented responses, and are more state-like than trait-like. These responses are free of intrasubjective self-references (e.g., "I hate myself because I always worry.") and are not global (e.g., "Everything makes me sad.").

Examples:
"I'm worried and nervous all the time."
"This pain is too much."
"I am sick of being depressed."

5. Global/General

This category refers to nonspecific, broad statements that are completely inclusive and therefore vague. These responses indicate a general, all-encompassing, or overarching sense of being overwhelmed and/or unable to cope.

Examples:
"The world around me."
"Life."
"Everything."

6. Situation-Specific

This category pertains to situation-specific responses (i.e., responses that speak to a certain place or time). Any reference made about a specific situation or circumstance, or any references made to a certain place, time, or events go here as well. (Note: A mention of a specific person would be better placed in the Relational category.)

Examples:
"When I come home to my empty apartment at night."
"First thing when I wake up."
"Whenever I hear a song by our favorite band."

7. Helpless

This category refers to implied or specific references to feeling out of control, lost, or trapped. References to feeling directionless are also in included in this category. General statements about hopelessness about one's inability to cope, function, or achieve in the future should be placed here. (If the statement refers to a role or responsibility [e.g., "My career"], place it in the Role/Responsibility category.)

Examples:
"Feeling so lost that I don't know where to go."
"I have no idea where I'm going."
"I will never amount to anything no matter what I do."

8. Unsure/Unable to Articulate

This category refers to responses in which the person is uncertain or unable to respond. It may include responses that seem purposely evasive, avoidant, or apathetic.

Examples:
"I don't know."
"I'm not saying."
"Who knows?"

AGITATION (PERTURBATION)

The Agitation SSF variable is based on Shneidman's (1993) construct of "perturbation." Perturbation is a Shneidman neologism that refers to a general term meaning the state of being upset or perturbed. In relation to suicide, perturbation includes (1) perceptual constriction, and (2) a penchant for precipitous self-harm or inimical action. Constriction refers to the reduction of an individual's perceptual and cognitive range. At its worst, constriction includes a narrow way of thinking, tunnel vision, and focusing on only a few options, with death and escape becoming the only solution to the problems of psychache and frustrated needs. A penchant for action refers to impulsivity, or a strong tendency to get things over with and come to quick resolution while having little patience and low tolerance for stressful situations. At its worst, there is a clear tendency toward precipitous and potentially impulsive self-destructive actions.

There is no other term in the suicidology literature that quite captures what Shneidman intends to describe by the term *perturbation*. Terms such as *anxiety, turmoil, impulsiveness, irritation,* or *annoyance* do not capture the cognitive and affective complexity inherent in the perturbation construct. Perhaps because of this, the construct can be elusive and difficult for both clinicians and patients to understand. In Luoma's (1999) study of SSF constructs, perturbation was one of the most difficult notions for undergraduates to grasp; their conceptual understanding tended to focus on negative emotions. This focus on negative emotions misses both the cognitively oriented perceptual constriction and the more affectivity oriented urgency or impulsiveness. Thus, building off this work the revised agitation SSF item was specifically defined as "emotional urgency; feeling that you need to take action; **not** irritation; **not** annoyance." Again, the revised definition only speaks to the emotional urgency side of the definition and does not speak to perceptual constriction per se. Finally, the stem used on the SSF form also includes a temporal component. Open-ended responses will therefore tend to be situation specific, because subjects are responding to the prompt, **"I need to take action when . . ."**

Coding Categories (Total of 9)

1. Compelled to Act

This category deals with a person's explicit desire to urgently change something in his or her life, a recognized need for a quick solution, a need to take action. Embedded in this category is an awareness of the lack of change (being stuck) and the need to do something decisive.

Examples:
"I just want to fix things now."
"I'm not doing anything."
"Something needs to be done to end this state I'm in."

2. Global/General

This category refers to nonspecific, broad statements that are completely inclusive and therefore vague. These responses indicate a general, all-encompassing, or overarching sense of being overwhelmed and/or unable to cope.

Examples:
"I feel utterly swamped."
"Everything comes down on me."
"My head is jumbled with all that I have to deal with."

3. Helpless

This category refers to explicit or implied statements regarding feeling out of control, lost, or unable to change things. References to feeling a loss of direction and not knowing about the future are also included in this category. References to constricted thinking, a lack of options, a narrow view of things as well as general statements about one's inability to cope, function, and achieve in the future should also be placed here.

Examples:
"Things are out of control."
"There is nothing I can do to make it better."
"I have no options, nothing will change."

4. Unsure/Unable to Articulate

This category refers to responses in which the person is uncertain or unable to respond. It may include responses that seem purposely evasive, avoidant, or apathetic.

Examples:
"Don't know."
"Unsure."
"Wouldn't you like to know?"

5. Situation-Specific

This category pertains to situation-specific responses (i.e., responses that speak to a certain place or time). Any reference made about a specific situation, circumstance, or any references made to a certain place, time, or events go here as well. (Note: A mention of a specific person would be better placed in the Relational category.)

Examples:
"I come home to my empty apartment at night."
"First thing when I wake up."
"I hear a song by our favorite band."

6. Unpleasant Internal States

This category refers to specific, discrete descriptions of hurting, distress, suffering, emotional pain, and other negative emotions in the mood spectrum. They are symptom-oriented responses, and are more state-like than trait-like. These responses are free of intrasubjective self-references (e.g., "I hate myself because I always worry.") and are not global (e.g., "Everything makes me sad.").

Examples:
"I feel anxious."
"I fall apart after I get angry."
"The depression is more than I can stand."

7. Self

This category refers to responses that are specific to one's self, or when a reference to one's self is clearly inferred. These can be statements about feelings or qualities about the self. These tend to include descriptions of enduring traits, core attributes, or harsh self-critiques or external descriptors about the self.

Examples:
"I see what a loser I am."
"I get particularly pathetic."
"I am such a mess, no one will love me."

8. Relational

This category refers to responses that make references to specific relationship problems or issues with children, spouse, partner, parents, friends, significant others, or any other social interaction. Any response that speaks to being hurt by others or hurting others goes here; specific references about being alone or isolated also go here.

Examples:
"Jim yells at me."
"I think about how I have no one who loves me in a romantic way."
"I disappoint my dad."

9. Role/Responsibilities

This category refers to responsibilities or obligations related to common adult role expectations, including the roles of the worker, homemaker, or student. Responses may be specific examples of a role or responsibility or an expression of feeling inefficient in these roles. Responses such as academic concerns, financial burdens, or job concerns are included here. Specific future-oriented statements regarding career are also included. Statements that refer to lack of direction or purpose should be placed in the Helpless category.

Examples:
"I think about how I have no idea what kind of job I want to get after school."
"I think about my future."
"I think about my finances."
"I can't decide on a job."
"I see how I suck at being a parent."

HOPELESSNESS

Hopelessness is a cognitive style rather than an emotional state; this distinction that makes hopelessness different from depression. Beck and colleagues (1979) refer to hopelessness as a set of beliefs an individual has that his or her situation will not improve regardless of what that individual does to change the situation. This set of beliefs can be focused on anything in an individual's life. It is theorized that individuals who believe their situation will never improve "give up" on life and lack desire to endure a situation they believe will never get better.

Hopelessness has been consistently found to be an important component of suicide risk and can be specifically addressed and modified in treatment (Brown, Beck, Steer, & Grisham, 2000). Hopelessness has also been proposed to be a construct that has different levels of conviction. For example, individuals who *think* their situation will not improve are at a lower risk for suicide than individuals who truly *believe* their situation will never get better.

Most measures of hopelessness tend to assess the global sense of the construct; however, more recent studies have emerged that are beginning to assess related constructs and components of hopelessness. For example, perfectionism is proposed to be a contributing factor to suicide risk. The theory is that individuals who set and maintain unrealistically high standards and expectations are at risk of suicide due to the fact that their standards are set so high that, in reality, they cannot achieve them. The individuals adopt a hopeless attitude because they will never be able to attain the personal or social expectations placed on them.

Other research suggests that hopeless individuals are unable to generate positive thoughts about the future or can only foresee negative events happening. These various theories and related constructs all have one common theme in tune with hopelessness: The individual does not believe a situation will improve regardless of what is done. Little work has been published on the specific areas that individuals find hopeless. Therefore, the stem used on the SSF form also includes a temporal component. Open-ended responses will therefore tend to be situation specific, because subjects are responding to the prompt **"I am most hopeless about . . ."**

Coding Categories (Total of 7)

1. General/Global

This category refers to nonspecific, broad statements that are completely inclusive and therefore vague. These responses indicate a general, all-encompassing, or overarching sense of being overwhelmed and/or unable to cope.

Examples:
"Life."
"Everything."
"Things in general."

2. Future

This category refers to broad statements or inferences about an individual's future. These statements can be *specific* or *nonspecific* statements about the future. Any global statements about the future would be placed in this category along with specific statement about any specific dreams, skills, events, or experiences (except career or school, see Role/Responsibilities) with a *clear reference to the future*.

Examples:
"The future."
"Achieving my dreams."
"Reaching my goals."

3. Relational

This category refers to responses that make references to specific relationship problems or issues with children, spouse, partner, parents, friends, significant others, or any other social interaction. Any response that speaks to being hurt by others or hurting others goes here; specific references about being alone or isolated also go here.

Examples:
"People at work."
"My relationship with my boyfriend."
"Everybody."

4. Role/Responsibilities

This category refers to responsibilities or obligations related to common adult role expectations, including the role of the worker, homemaker, or student. Responses may be specific examples of a role or responsibility or may be an expression of feeling inefficient in these roles. Responses such as academic concerns, financial burdens, or job concerns are included here. These responses can be broad references in the present about getting things done. Specific future-oriented statements regarding career are also included.

Examples:
"Achieving my career ambitions."
"Getting done with school."
"Money."

5. Self

This category refers to responses that are specific to one's self, or when a reference to one's self is clearly inferred. These can be statements about feelings or qualities about the self. These tend to include descriptions of enduring traits, core attributes or harsh self-critiques or external descriptors about the self. Statements about gaining control of one's behavior, thoughts, or feelings would be included in this category.

Examples:
"Understanding myself."
"Being too fat."
"I'm bad at dealing with my emotions."

6. Unpleasant Internal States

This category refers to specific, discrete descriptions of hurting, distress, suffering, emotional pain, and other negative emotions in the mood spectrum. They are symptom-oriented responses, and are more state-like than trait-like. These responses are free of intrasubjective self-references (e.g., "I hate myself because I always worry.") and are not global (e.g., "Everything makes me sad.").

Examples:
"My anxiety will never go away."
"How I fall apart after I get angry."
"I am afraid I will always be depressed."

7. Unsure/Unable to Articulate

This category refers to responses in which the person is uncertain or unable to respond. It may include responses that seem purposely evasive, avoidant, or apathetic.

Examples:
"Don't know."
"Not sure."
"Who cares?"

SELF-HATE

Self-hate can be conceptualized as the negative affect that proceeds from an increase in self-awareness (Baumeister, 1990). The individual experiences an event that falls short of personal standards and/or expectations. Consequently, when internal attributions are made to explain that event, one begins to hate the self and seeks to diminish this state through cognitive deconstruction. The deconstruction lowers thought processes and inhibitions, making a suicide attempt more likely.

Typically individuals have a preferred view of the self, which is supported and maintained by various psychological mechanisms. When these views are challenged (especially in the context of therapy) the patient may witness the "dreaded sense of self" as opposed to the former "ideal self." Such a transition often leads to self-hate and can act as a trigger for a suicide attempt (Baumeister, 1990).

Finally, self-hate can be conceptualized as a cycle. The idea is that an individual engages in self-detrimental actions due to self-hate. The negative consequences of such actions lead to an increase in self-hate, which may become a cycle. The individual may then either downgrade achievements to confirm to an initial view of the self (high achievement self-hate) or strive less in order to justify potential failures. Therefore, the stem **"What I hate most about myself is . . ."** is included to further elucidate a suicidal person's experience of self-hate.

Coding Categories (Total of 7)

1. Helpless

This category refers to explicit or implied statements regarding feeling out of control, lost, or unable to change things. References to feeling a loss of direction and not knowing about the future are also included in this category. References to constricted thinking, a lack of options, a narrow view of things as well as general statements about ones inability to cope, function, and achieve in the future should also be placed here.

Examples:
"I'm not able to talk about my problem."
"I have no way of stopping my depression."
"I have nowhere to go from here."

2. Internal Descriptors

This category refers to statements about an individual's lack of positive qualities or the presence of negative qualities in him- or herself. These can also be statements about feelings about the self and tend to include harsh self-critiques about inner descriptors of the self.

Examples:
"I'm a coward."
"I'm not intelligent."
"I'm a mess all the time."

3. External Descriptors

This category refers to statements about how an individual dislikes some external, outer aspect of him- or herself such as his or her personal appearance, body, or behaviors he or she is engaging in.

Examples:
"My drug use."
"I always look ugly."
"My body."

4. Relational

This category refers to responses that make references to specific relationship problems or issues with children, spouse, partner, parents, friends, significant others, or any other social interaction. Any response that speaks to being hurt by others or hurting others goes here; specific references about being alone or isolated also go here as well.

Examples:
"Hurting my parents."
"My girlfriend broke up with me."
"I can't fit in here at school."

5. Global/General

This category refers to nonspecific, broad statements that are completely inclusive and therefore vague. These responses indicate a general, all-encompassing, or overarching sense of being dissatisfied with life in general and/or overwhelmed.

Examples:
"Everything about me I hate."
"Myself."
"My entire life."

6. Role/Responsibilities

This category refers to statements about responsibilities or obligations related to common adult role expectations including the role of the worker, homemaker, or student. Responses may be specific examples of a role or responsibility or may be an expression of feeling inefficient in these roles. Responses such as academic concerns, financial burdens, or job concerns are included here. Specific future-oriented statements regarding career are also included. Statements that refer to lack of direction or purpose should be placed in the Helpless category.

Examples:
"I can't make enough money."
"I can't decide on a job."
"I suck at being a parent."

7. Unsure/Unable to Articulate

This category refers to responses in which the person is uncertain or unable to respond. It may include responses that seem purposely evasive, avoidant, or apathetic.

Examples:
"Don't know."
"Can't say."
"You tell me."

APPENDIX C

Coding Manual for SSF Reasons
for Living versus Reasons for Dying

CODING MANUAL:
DECATEGORIZATION OF REASONS FOR LIVING AND REASONS FOR DYING

OVERVIEW

Past empirical and theoretical work in the area of suicidology has focused primarily on two separate and diametrically opposite areas; risk factors and motivations for suicide (Reasons for Dying), and life-sustaining beliefs (Reasons for Living). These two bodies of research have provided rich and useful insight into the motivations for suicide. However, to more fully understand an individual's suicidal motivation requires a more comprehensive, balanced consideration: what sustains one's life versus what makes one want to give up? Perhaps examining both reasons for living *and* reasons for dying together may enable us to better understand the significance of both sides of the suicidal equation.

WHY REASONS FOR LIVING AND DYING?

Linehan and colleagues (1983) believed that suicidal individuals lacked life-oriented beliefs that would keep them from committing suicide. They developed the Reasons for Living Inventory to measure how important these beliefs are for not committing suicide. Six factors were identified as sets of reasons for living: Survival and Coping, Responsibility to Family, Child-Related Concerns, Fear of Suicide, Fear of Social Disapproval, and Moral Objections. However, the information gleaned from the Reasons for Living Inventory only contributes to one side of the equation. It is also important to understand an individual's motivation to commit suicide and what factors exist in place of the beliefs for living. This is why it is important to ask for reasons for dying as well. This line of thinking led to the development of the RFL versus RFD assessment in order to formally study the full suicidal equation. In an effort to better understand the suicidal mind, individuals who expressed feelings of suicidality were asked to list their RFL and their RFD. The individuals were asked to organize each list in order of importance.

Superordinate Categories

Jobes and Mann (1999) showed that the RFL and RFD can be organized into meaningfully different reliable coding categories. One purpose of the current coding process is to further organize the categories into larger, more inclusive superordinate categories: hopefulness for self, others, and future, and hopelessness for self, others, and future.

Hopefulness and Hopelessness for Self, Others, and the Future

According to Beck's (1967) cognitive theory of depression, depressed individuals express a negative view of themselves, their world, and their future. This is the "negative triad" or the "cognitive triad." These negative views are often translated into feelings and expressions of hopelessness or negative expectations. Beck (1986) discussed that feelings of hopelessness are one of the single best predictors of suicidality as well as an excellent indicator of current suicidal intent. In contrast to hopelessness as a risk factor for suicidality, hopefulness can be considered a protective factor against it. Range and Penton (1994) found that RFL are positively correlated with hope and negatively correlated with hopelessness.

Self and Other

Bakan (1966) used the terms *agency* and *communion* to indicate the poles of a continuum for human experience. Agency signifies the desire for individuation, self-protection, and self-direction. Communion signifies the desire for personal relationships, attachment and intimacy. Each individual falls somewhere on this continuum. This notion of agency and communion can be built on when attempting to understand the suicidal individual. Jobes (1995) described this continuum using the terms *intrapsychic* (self) and *interpsychic* (other). The intrapsychic pole of the continuum would be defined by a concentration on internal, subjective, phenomenological issues. The suicidal individual who would be described as being intrapsychic would focus primarily on issues pertaining to the self rather than to others. At the opposite end of the continuum, the interpsychic pole would be understood as a concentration on external, relational issues. In this case, the suicidal individual would focus predominantly on others and interpersonal relationships rather than on the self.

Connecting Categories to Superordinate Categories

To determine which categories would fit into each of the superordinate categories, an addendum to the coding manual would need to be developed and tested for interrater reliability. However, theory and common sense can be applied to make assumptions about which superordinate category each category would fall in. Based on the literature on motivations for suicide and life-sustaining beliefs, RFL should be placed in the overarching category of Hopefulness, and RFD should be placed in Hopelessness. The RFL categories Enjoyable Things, Beliefs, and Self would fall under the heading of Hopefulness about the Self. The RFL categories Family, Friends, Responsibility to Others, and Burdening Others would fall under the heading of Hopefulness about Others. The remaining RFL categories Hopefulness for the Future and Plans and Goals would fall under the heading of Hopefulness for the Future. Likewise, the RFD categories of Loneliness, General Descriptors of Self, and the Escape categories would fall under the heading of Hopelessness about the Self. The RFD categories of Others (Relationships) and Unburdening Others would fall under the category of Hopelessness about Others. The RFD category of Hopelessness would clearly fall under the heading of Hopelessness about the Future.

GENERAL GUIDELINES FOR CODING

Coders will be given actual responses from the lists made by the suicidal clients on RFL and RFD. Clients typically listed up to five responses for each list. Each response is provided in its own line of a coding sheet. There are two separate sets of coding sheets, one for RFL and one for RFD. Each set of responses should be coded independently of one the other. The categories within a set should be considered as mutually exclusive of one another. Therefore, each reason should only be placed into *one* category and subsequently given *one* code. When coding a reason, although some interpretation may be necessary, the coder should generally take the response at face value and do as little guesswork as possible into the motivations and/or circumstances that might surround the reason.

Specific Guidelines for Coding

The category labels are located at the top of the columns on the right side of the coding sheets. The coders are given the collection of responses for that set. Coders are to make a determination about which category the response should be placed into and put a checkmark in the appropriate category column. Before proceeding to the next response, the coder should rate from 1 to 5 the confidence of his or her choice in the Confidence Rating column. The rating is made on a scale from 1 to 5, 1 being "not confident at all" and 5 being "highly confident." Once the response has been placed in a category and the confidence rating has been completed, the coder should then move to the next response. After completing these tasks for one set of responses, the coder should repeat the process for the other set of responses.

WHAT ARE THE CODINGS USED FOR?

There are two purposes for coding the RFL/RFD assessment responses. The first is to identify common categories into which these reasons might fall. The second is to use these categorized responses to develop types of suicidal individuals that can predict treatment outcomes.

Reasons for Living Coding Categories

1. Family

This category deals with any references to family such as marriage or children.

> **Examples:**
> "My parents."
> "My parents love me."
> "My husband."
> "My fiancé."

2. Friends

This category refers to any mention of friends including specific names (e.g., John or Cindy). References to a boyfriend or girlfriend should also be placed in this category. If the response indicates that the person referred to is a family member, then place in the family category.

Note: If both family and friends are mentioned in the same response, place it in the category of the first group that is identified. For example, if the response says "family and friends," then place this response in the family category, but if the response reads "friends and family," place it in the friends category.

3. Responsibility to Others

This category deals with responses that have to do with responsibilities and obligations owed to other people.

> **Examples:**
> "Working in the bookstore."
> "I don't want to disappoint people."

4. Burdening Others

This category refers to statements regarding concerns, fears, or anxieties around troubling or burdening others (family, friends, other specifically identified individuals) with the aftermath of their suicide.

> **Examples:**
> "Family guilt." or "I don't want to upset anyone."
> "My parents would be really upset if I died."
> "Father Brian would be very upset if I killed myself."

5. Plans and Goals

This category deals with statements referring to future-oriented plans. The statements may express a desire to see something through or to deal with things that are left to be completed. These are typically self-oriented statements. However, they should be placed in this category when referring to goals or future plans. These statements contain a sense of action. More general "self" referencing statements should be placed in the Self category, category 9.

> **Examples:**
> "I want to finish school." or "I want to travel to Europe."
> "I want to have children someday."
> "There is still so much that I want to do with my life."

6. Hopefulness for the Future

This category refers to future-oriented statements that deal with vague abstract yearnings. The statements express a hopeful attitude or refer to a curiosity of how things are going to turn out, but are more passive than those statements falling in the category of Plans and Goals, category 5.

Examples:
"My dreams."
"I think things will work out." or "I hope I will stop feeling bad."
"I want to find out what is going to happen."

7. Enjoyable Things

This category refers to activities or objects that are merely mentioned or are referred to as something that is enjoyed. These references also include objects of value like a pet or a possession.

Examples:
"Chinese food."
"Playing the piano." or "Music."
"My cat."

8. Beliefs

This category deals with responses referring to religion, personal beliefs, or ethics. These responses may include but are not limited to references to God or another religious figure. If the statement refers to a specified religious figure in the context of burdening this individual, then this statement should be place in the Burdening Others category, category 3.

Examples:
"It is a sin." or "I want to be able to go to heaven."

9. Self

This category deals with references specific to the self or when the reference to self is clearly inferred. These include references to feelings or qualities about the self. The responses can also be references to owing oneself something. These are not future-oriented statements. If the statements make references to the future, they should be placed in either the Plans and Goals or Hopefulness for the Future categories (category 5 or 6).

Examples:
"Myself."
"I don't think I could go through with it."
"I don't want to let myself down."
"I'm not that kind of person."

Reasons for Dying Coding Categories

1. Others (Relationships)

This category deals with references to other people, both explicitly and inferred.

Examples:
"To see my mother in heaven."
"Retribution."

2. Unburdening Others

This category refers to suicide as a solution for ending the hardship that the individual believes he or she causes other people.

Examples:
"To stop hurting others."
"To not cause anyone else stress."
"Relieve the financial burden on my family."
"I am afraid of hurting people I care about."

3. Loneliness

This category refers to statements about loneliness.

Examples:
"I don't want to be lonely anymore."
"Feeling alone."
"I don't have anyone."
"I have no one to talk to."

4. Hopelessness

This category refers to statements about hopelessness about the future.

Examples:
"Things may never get better." or "I don't think things will work out."
"I'm afraid I'll never reach my goals." or "I'm never going to amount to anything."
"Things may never get better between me and my girlfriend."
"I'm depressed that things will never change."

5. General Descriptors of Self

This category deals with feelings about the self as well as general references to the self.

Examples:
"Myself."
"I'm not worth anything."
"Worried."
"I feel awful."
"I will always feel this way."

Note: The next several categories deal with the issue of escape. Escape refers to a statement dealing with a need or desire to get away from or end something. The "something" could be a feeling, an obligation, or an event.

6. Escape—In General

This category refers to general statement about escape as well as references to a general attitude of giving up.

Examples:

"I want to find peace." or ""I can't take it anymore."
"Escape." or "There would be less stress."
"I need a rest." or "To end my life." or "Life sucks."

7. Escape—The Past

This category deals with statements generally referring to the past or getting away from past experiences and feelings.

Examples:

"My childhood was not fun." or "I would like to start over."
"I want to break from my past."

8. Escape—The Pain

This category refers to specific statements about psychological pain and the desire to stop the pain.

Examples:

"I don't want to feel pain anymore."
"No more pain."
"I want to stop the hurt, the ache."

9. Escape—Responsibilities

This category deals with statements making references to getting out of responsibilities.

Examples:

"I don't want to be responsible anymore."
"To not be responsible."
"I hate working in the bookstore."

Coding Manual for the SSF
One-Thing Response

THE SSF "ONE-THING" CODING MANUAL

OVERVIEW

The Suicide Status Form (SSF; Jobes et al., 1997) is a suicide risk assessment instrument that attempts to measure a client's suicidality from both a quantitative and qualitative standpoint. This coding manual will be used to analyze qualitative data derived from a specific assessment construct of the SSF, namely, the "One-Thing" Response. In this assessment suicidal clients are prompted to provide a written answer to the following question: **"The one thing that will help me no longer feel suicidal is . . ."** This manual employs three conceptual dimensions (Orientation; Reality Testing; Clinical Utility) in an attempt to reliably group various written open-ended responses to the "One-Thing" assessment.

The purpose of the coding task is to further test and refine the SSF to establish it as a valid and reliable suicide risk assessment instrument. In particular, the codings for the "One-Thing" Response will help clinicians and researchers understand an important facet of a client's suicidality, namely, the one thing that may make a difference in terms of potential suicide risk.

GENERAL GUIDELINES FOR CODING

Step 1

Coders will receive a pack of index cards. Each card depicts one client's answer to the "One-Thing" prompt. The coders will be asked to make an <u>initial</u> sort and rate each response according to the three conceptual dimensions:

1. Orientation (Self vs. Relational vs. Not Codable)
2. Reality Testing (Realistic vs. Unrealistic vs. Not Codable)
3. Clinical Utility (Clinically Relevant Information vs. No Clinically Relevant Information vs. Not Codable)

The three choices for each coding dimension are mutually exclusive; hence, a response cannot be both "self" and "others." Each response should be coded in terms of these three coding dimensions and should thus have three coding responses.

Example:

"I want to have a better relationship with my peers."

1. Orientation (Others)
2. Reality Testing (Realistic)
3. Clinical Utility (Clinically Relevant Information)

Step 2

After the initial sort, a <u>second</u> sort will be performed to make sure that the coders are comfortable with their choices. In order that we may better understand the decision making process, the coders should discuss the rationale behind their specific coding. In addition, the coders should rate their confidence in the coding they have made for each particular response. The confidence levels are as follows:

1 = indicates a low level of confidence
2 = indicates a medium level of confidence
3 = indicates a high level of confidence

CODING DEFINITIONS AND EXAMPLES

Coding Dimension One: The Orientation of the Person's Response

Self

This category refers to anything about <u>the self</u>: It can be something that the person does/does not, feels/feels not, thinks/thinks not, or descriptions that are self-referential.

Examples:

> "To like myself better."
> "To be less depressed."
> "To no longer have these sad feelings."
> "Obtain a better grade in class."
> "Find more interests and be more confident."
> "Go away for a while."

Relational

This category refers to anything about <u>others or relationships</u>: It can be any social relationship (family, coworkers, romantic, etc.) and it can be either an existing relationship, an old relationship, or lack of a relationship.

Examples:

> "To have Jim love me again."
> "To have someone who I can talk to who understands me."
> "Somehow having more/better friends."
> "Relief from memories of parental abuse."
> "Seeing my mom again who died."
> "Problems with boyfriend."

Not Codable

In this category, there is no content to the answer or no answer at all: <u>It does not</u> receive further coding on the other two dimensions.

Examples:

> "Don't know."
> "How should I know?"
> "Who cares?"
> "I'm no longer suicidal."

Coding Dimension Two: The Reality Testing of the Person's Response

Realistic

This category refers to any item that can theoretically be obtained or that has a high probability of being achieved.

Examples:

"To have good friends."
"To have someone to talk to."
"To feel confident."
"Date more often with nice men."
"To pass my exams."
"To one day have a great family."

Unrealistic

This category refers to any item that is theoretically impossible, or not likely to be obtained/achieved.

Examples:

"To be free of all stress."
"Not to have been raped—undo the past."
"No thinking, no feeling, no worrying about things."
"A modern-day miracle."

Not Codable

There is no content to the answer or no answer at all; it does not receive further coding on the other two dimensions

Examples:

"Don't know."
"How should I know?"
"Who cares?"
"I'm no longer suicidal."

Coding Dimension Three: The Clinical Utility of the Person's Response

Clinically Relevant Information

This category refers to any comments that identify new information related to a starting point for therapy or the use of a specific therapeutic technique. In other words, does the response guide or shape possible clinical interventions?

Examples:

"Do better in school." (academic skills)
"To rebuild a relationship with X." (social skills)
"To date more often." (social skills)
"To have good friends." (social skills)
"To not have been abused." (abuse issues)
"Less stress." (progressive relaxation)

No Clinically Relevant Information

This category refers to any item that is vague or requests the help of resolving suicidality, or is not addressable by clinical intervention.

Examples:

> "To be reborn as a man."
> "To win a million dollars."
> "To marry Madonna."

Not Codable

In this category there is no content to the answer or no answer at all: <u>It does not</u> receive further coding on the other two dimensions

Examples:

> "Don't know."
> "How should I know?"
> "Who cares?"
> "I'm no longer suicidal"

SPECIFIC GUIDELINES AND DECISION RULES FOR CODING

The coders should use the manual as needed during the coding process. This section is designed to provide coding guidance and certain decision rules for uncertain codings. At least three possible coding dilemmas may arise in relation to coding "One-Thing" Responses.

Dilemma 1: Multiple Responses

Might occur in any of the three dimensions.

Example:

> "To not be so stressed, to have more dates, for this semester to be over."

> 1. Orientation   (Self)
> 2. Reality Testing   (Realistic)
> 3. Clinical Utility   (Clinically Relevant Direction)

If two or more answers are identified, a decision rule is to use the <u>first response</u> in a string of responses. In this case, the answer is "to not be so stressed."

Dilemma 2: Specificity versus Broad Concept

Occurs only in the Reality Testing Dimension. The coders should take these statements at face value without any attempt to philosophize about the details of the statement. For example, it could be that a client has a restraining order against them. In the second example, it could be that the client has nowhere to live or has no means to live in California. In the third example, the client might not be able to find another job. All this does not matter for the present purpose. The task is to rate whether a given response is obtainable in <u>a rather broad manner</u>. If a statement has any chance of being fulfilled it is to be coded as realistic. All of the foregoing examples would be realistic.

Examples:

"To get back with my boyfriend Jim."
"To go back home to California."
"To get another job, a more fulfilling one."

Dilemma 3: Unrealistic but Clinically Relevant

Occurs only in the Clinical Utility Dimension.

Example:

"To be free of all stress."

This would be coded as "unrealistic" insofar as it is not theoretically possible. However, it has clinical utility (Clinically Relevant Information) because it tells us that the client has a difficulty with stress and possibly in dealing with stress. Thus, a Reality Testing "Unrealistic" rating <u>does not</u> necessarily imply a clinical utility "No Clinically Relevant Information" rating. In other words, simply because a response is unrealistic (theoretically impossible) does not mean that it is not clinically useful.

THE SSF "ONE-THING" CODING SHEET

Client ID	Orientation	Reality Testing	Clinical Utility
	Self ____ Other ____ Not Codable ____ C.L. 1 2 3	Realistic ____ Unrealistic ____ Not Codable ____ C.L. 1 2 3	Provides Clinically Relevant Info ____ Provides No Clinically Relevant Info ____ Not Codable ____ C.L. 1 2 3
	Self ____ Other ____ Not Codable ____ C.L. 1 2 3	Realistic ____ Unrealistic ____ Not Codable ____ C.L. 1 2 3	Provides Clinically Relevant Info ____ Provides No Clinically Relevant Info ____ Not Codable ____ C.L. 1 2 3
	Self ____ Other ____ Not Codable ____ C.L. 1 2 3	Realistic ____ Unrealistic ____ Not Codable ____ C.L. 1 2 3	Provides Clinically Relevant Info ____ Provides No Clinically Relevant Info ____ Not Codable ____ C.L. 1 2 3
	Self ____ Other ____ Not Codable ____ C.L. 1 2 3	Realistic ____ Unrealistic ____ Not Codable ____ C.L. 1 2 3	Provides Clinically Relevant Info ____ Provides No Clinically Relevant Info ____ Not Codable ____ C.L. 1 2 3
	Self ____ Other ____ Not Codable ____ C.L. 1 2 3	Realistic ____ Unrealistic ____ Not Codable ____ C.L. 1 2 3	Provides Clinically Relevant Info ____ Provides No Clinically Relevant Info ____ Not Codable ____ C.L. 1 2 3
	Self ____ Other ____ Not Codable ____ C.L. 1 2 3	Realistic ____ Unrealistic ____ Not Codable ____ C.L. 1 2 3	Provides Clinically Relevant Info ____ Provides No Clinically Relevant Info ____ Not Codable ____ C.L. 1 2 3
	Self ____ Other ____ Not Codable ____ C.L. 1 2 3	Realistic ____ Unrealistic ____ Not Codable ____ C.L. 1 2 3	Provides Clinically Relevant Info ____ Provides No Clinically Relevant Info ____ Not Codable ____ C.L. 1 2 3
	Self ____ Other ____ Not Codable ____ C.L. 1 2 3	Realistic ____ Unrealistic ____ Not Codable ____ C.L. 1 2 3	Provides Clinically Relevant Info ____ Provides No Clinically Relevant Info ____ Not Codable ____ C.L. 1 2 3
	Self ____ Other ____ Not Codable ____ C.L. 1 2 3	Realistic ____ Unrealistic ____ Not Codable ____ C.L. 1 2 3	Provides Clinically Relevant Info ____ Provides No Clinically Relevant Info ____ Not Codable ____ C.L. 1 2 3
	Self ____ Other ____ Not Codable ____ C.L. 1 2 3	Realistic ____ Unrealistic ____ Not Codable ____ C.L. 1 2 3	Provides Clinically Relevant Info ____ Provides No Clinically Relevant Info ____ Not Codable ____ C.L. 1 2 3

APPENDIX E

Frequently Asked Questions about CAMS

FAQS ABOUT CAMS

Question: There is so much paperwork with CAMS, is it okay to use just parts of the SSF and not necessarily all the forms?

Answer: Yes, there is a lot of paperwork, but it is important to remember that extensive and thorough documentation of assessment and treatment is the most protective thing you can have on your side in cases of malpractice liability. Having said that, I know that many clinicians use only certain portions of the SSF. For example, some clinicians use only the assessment portions (A and B) of the first two pages of the index session SSF; others do not like to use the HIPAA pages preferring the use of other documentation. Throughout this book I have endeavored to emphasize the flexible and adaptable nature of CAMS and SSF use. In this sense, I am genuinely interested in clinicians using any or all of the materials as they see fit. Obviously from my own bias, however, using CAMS as I have outlined it in this book makes the most sense from both a clinical treatment and liability standpoint.

Question: Can I continue to track a Suicide Status case even though the patient meets the criteria for resolution?

Answer: Yes, of course. I know a number of clinicians who prefer to continue tracking Suicide Status cases even though they technically meet the CAMS resolution criteria described in this book because they do not trust that the patient is truly "out of the woods" in relation to suicide. This practice is up to the discretion of the clinician. Frankly, I think there is no particular downside to erring on the side of continuing ongoing monitoring. For example, at Johns Hopkins Counseling Center, where we have done a great deal of research, we see clinicians there routinely continuing to track cases even though we (the researchers) feel that a case should be considered "resolved." While ongoing tracking is fine, I personally like to formally resolve my Suicide Status cases as a meaningful landmark in the course of our clinical work together. In fact I actually make a big deal of the patient's resolving Suicide Status, using it as an opportunity to reflect on how far things have come and to reinforce the patient's sense of therapeutic success.

Question: How hard should I push to get other people in the patient's life involved in the Crisis Response Plan?

Answer: As with all clinical decision making, it depends on the case. I am very preoccupied with the importance of trying to engage supportive others. Of course, this must be done with a signed release by the patient. Some patients are very reluctant to get others involved; alternatively, other patients seem quite comfortable with the concept. It is perhaps more important to have at least considered the potential value of engaging significant others. In other words, if you ultimately judge that it is not in the patient's best interest to engage others, it is still important to document your clinical decision making about this professional judgment.

Question: When is a patient too young for CAMS?

Answer: The youngest patient I have used this approach with was 12. I would think, however, that CAMS could be used with children as young as 6 or 8 years old. In such cases, the clinician may need to take a much more active and directive role in explaining the SSF constructs in language that the child can appreciate and understand. The same holds for patients with cognitive limitations. As long as one can be patient and work to clarify SSF constructs in a more deliberative manner, there is no reason that CAMS cannot be used with a broad range of suicidal patients.

Question: What if the patient refuses to have you take an adjacent seat?

Answer: There are certain cases in which physical boundary issues may necessarily prohibit the adjacent seating arrangement recommended in CAMS. A patient's refusal to have you switch seats must be understood and respected as legitimate and you should never force the issue. In such cases, CAMS can proceed in a face-to-face manner passing the clipboard back and forth at the transition points. I am very sensitive to the therapeutic value of adjacent seating and the potential for discomfort. For example, in my office I personally do not feel comfortable sitting on the love seat, which would place me directly beside the patient—it is just too close. Instead, I pull up my desk chair and place it adjacent to the patient at an angle that enables us to work together comfortably.

Question: I have a case that I have worked with for some years. We are totally stuck and the issue of suicide has been contentious in our work. Can I really introduce CAMS at this point with any hope of it being helpful?

Answer: Yes, you can. I have three long-term cases in which a significant overhaul of the treatment plan was absolutely necessary, particularly in relation to the issue of suicide. I would suggest introducing the idea of needing to reexamine the treatment from top to bottom. In this regard, you can propose a new approach (CAMS), which might actually give the two of you a fresh start and the potential to grapple with the issue of suicide perhaps differently than you have previously. I often receive feedback from clinicians who have gone to one of my workshop trainings who proceed to try CAMS with just this type of case. They often report back to me that the patient was intrigued and engaged by CAMS. Moreover, these long term patients often express appreciation for the clinician's effort to "reboot" the treatment.

Complete CAMS Case Example

COMPLETE CAMS CASE EXAMPLE: STEVE JOHNSON

The following is complete CAMS case example of "Steve Johnson." Steve was a 24-year-old newly graduated engineer referred to me by a colleague working at a university counseling center. Steve had been seen by the referring clinician for three crisis sessions in late May, 2 weeks prior to his graduation when he would receive a master's degree in engineering. He presented to me in a highly distressed state—clearly distraught over his having no job, and a pervasive sense of being lost, isolated, and notably depressed. He cried on and off throughout our first session and readily acknowledged thoughts of suicide. His OQ-45 revealed significant symptom distress and "frequent" thoughts of suicide. Specifically, he was preoccupied with jumping off a particularly high bridge in Washington, DC.

I noted his level of distress and within the first 10 minutes took a seat adjacent to Steve as we began to complete the index SSF. As can be seen on page 191, the patient has high ratings of pain and hopelessness as well as an overall behavioral risk of "3." He had reasonable Reasons for Living; Reasons for Dying focused on escape and worries about the future. His One-Thing Response on the SSF focused on work and love.

On page 192 we see some worrisome suicidal ideation with a specific plan and history of suicidal thoughts dating back to teenage years. He was very focused on a bridge that he routinely crossed and had even considered the best location from which to jump. He had passing thoughts of going home (Boston) to get his father's rifle but did not seriously consider this a viable option. In terms of other risk variables, his history of ideation is a concern but there was never an actual attempt. He was preoccupied still with a previous girlfriend who had ended their relationship the preceding fall. He had significant issues with his family of origin—particularly his father—and there was considerable shame connected to his family and father. Bottom line, he was very open to psychotherapy and wanted to be motivated but he largely thought he was a "lost cause."

In terms of the treatment plan, he was clear about not wanting to go to the hospital. I used this fear as leverage to focus on an intensive outpatient plan that included twice-a-week meetings and a referral to a psychiatrist for possible medication. In terms of the Crisis Response Plan, we developed a Crisis Card together and he committed to taking a different walking route avoiding the bridge and to reading the book *Choosing to Live* by Tom Ellis and Corey Newman. We identified two other problems for his treatment plan: his unemployment and social isolation, which he felt were the problems at the heart of his current crisis.

The HIPAA form [on page 193] of the SSF notes a very distressed and depressed/anxious patient. The mental status exam revealed that the patient was oriented with no evidence of psychosis. There was evidence of marked dysphoria with labile affect. The patient was diagnosed (provisionally) with an adjustment disorder with depressed and anxious mood; Global Assessment of Functioning was only a 50, reflecting serious impairment. The overall formulation of suicidal risk was moderate risk—there was no clear and imminent danger in my view, mostly due to the patient's notable willingness to work on an intensive outpatient basis and his commitment to trying the Crisis Card and other coping approaches.

As can be seen by the SSF Tracking forms, the case progressed rather nicely. After the index session, there were a total of five Suicide Status sessions as the patient conscientiously followed our treatment plan. He was able to quickly see my consulting psychiatrist and began Prozac almost immediately after our initial session. He religiously used his Coping Card and never felt the need to ultimately call me. A key factor in his work was his journal writing, which he did extensively. As can be seen, there were some modifications in the treatment plan as we progressed. In our second session we added the problem of depression and anxiety, as he felt gradually better able to reach out to others for support. He also got his unemployment issue into a better perspective. With a loan from his mother (without his father knowing), he was able to be less frantic and thereby was better able to focus on a reasonable job hunt that could last for the balance of the summer. With the press of finding a job immediately removed, he felt much better overall and developed a thoughtful plan for systematically pursing various job options.

A key development within the first weeks was his increased involvement with a female roommate who was herself in therapy and very supportive of Steve. This relationship blossomed into a romance, which was very affirming to Steve. There was, however, a crisis after they first started dating that briefly set him back, but they worked things out and the relationship became a major source of happiness and support. Within the first weeks of taking the medication, we saw a clear therapeutic response—he felt more energized and described a "dark veil" being removed from his eyes.

Suicidal thinking began to wane after only a handful of sessions. Steve found that a synergy of changes orchestrated in our CAMS work together were cumulatively having a positive impact. Within a total of seven sessions, his suicidal ideation had completely disappeared and we resolved his Suicide Status with great mutual satisfaction.

With suicide no longer a coping option for Steve, we proceeded to work together on a once-per-week basis for 3 more years. Most of that work centered around some serious family-of-origin issues, which were very painful but important to address. After our first 6 months Steve found an excellent job. He dated his former roommate for about 2 years but they ultimately parted ways. Steve excelled professionally and found a sequence of jobs that placed him at the top of his field. He e-mailed me a couple of years ago to inform me that he had married and he was looking forward to starting a family with his new wife.

In our termination session Steve sincerely thanked me for "saving my life." Although it is tempting to personally take that kind of credit, I believe that I was the right person, at the right time, with the right knowledge, and an approach—CAMS—that made the difference. CAMS helped us create a treatment trajectory that made it clear to Steve that by collaboratively working together, we could indeed find a way to help him realize a life that was truly worth living.

SUICIDE STATUS FORM–III (SSF III) INITIAL SESSION

Patient: _____ Clinician: _____ Date: _____ Time: _____

Section A (Patient):

Rank — Rate and fill out each item according to how you feel <u>right now</u>.
Then rank items in order of importance 1 to 5 (1 = most important to 5 = least important).

Rank	
2	1) **RATE PSYCHOLOGICAL PAIN** (*hurt, anguish, or misery in your mind;* ***not*** *stress;* ***not*** *physical pain*): **Low Pain: 1 2 3 4 ⑤ :High Pain** What I find most painful is: *no job, isolated*
4	2) **RATE STRESS** (*your general feeling of being pressured or overwhelmed*): **Low Stress: 1 2 3 ④ 5 :High Stress** What I find most stressful is: *uncertain about future*
5	3) **RATE AGITATION** (*emotional urgency; feeling that you need to take action;* ***not*** *irritation;* ***not*** *annoyance*): **Low Agitation: 1 2 ③ 4 5 :High Agitation** I most need to take action when: *at night, when I go to bed*
1	4) **RATE HOPELESSNESS** (*your expectation that things will not get better no matter what you do*): **Low Hopelessness: 1 2 3 4 ⑤ :High Hopelessness** I am most hopeless about: *everything, things never work out for me*
3	5) **RATE SELF-HATE** (*your general feeling of disliking yourself; having no self-esteem; having no self-respect*): **Low Self-Hate: 1 2 3 ④ 5 :High Self-Hate** What I hate most about myself is: *being lost again*
N/A	6) **RATE OVERALL RISK OF SUICIDE:** **Extremely Low Risk: 1 2 ③ 4 5 :Extremely High Risk** **(will not kill self) (will kill self)**

1) How much is being suicidal related to thoughts and feelings about <u>yourself</u>? **Not at all: 1 2 3 4 ⑤ :completely**
2) How much is being suicidal related to thoughts and feelings about <u>others</u>? **Not at all: ① 2 3 4 5 :completely**

Please list your reasons for wanting to live and your reasons for wanting to die. Then rank in order of importance 1 to 5.

Rank	REASONS FOR LIVING	Rank	REASONS FOR DYING
3	my intelligence	2	things never work out
1	a good job	1	can't take the pain
2	finding someone to love	3	won't find healthy relationship
4	my brother	4	I hate myself like this

I wish to live to the following extent: Not at all: 0   1   2   3   ④   5   6   7   8 :Very much
I wish to die to the following extent: Not at all: 0   1   2   3   ④   5   6   7   8 :Very much

The one thing that would help me no longer feel suicidal would be: *to find a job and a good relationship*

SUICIDE STATUS FORM–III INITIAL SESSION (PAGE 2)

Section B (*Clinician*):

(Y) N Suicide Plan:

When: _not sure_

Where: _jump off bridge_

How: _jump_   **(Y)** N Access to means

How: _maybe use rifle_   Y **(N)** Access to means
(not now)

(Y) N Suicide Preparation   Describe: _wrote note to brother_

(Y) N Suicide Rehearsal   Describe: _picked spot on bridge to jump_

(Y) N History of Suicidality

    • Ideation   Describe: _as a teen had significant suicidal thoughts_

      • Frequency   _1–2_ per day _____ per week _____ per month

now   • Duration   _____ seconds _30_ minutes _1_ hours

      • Single Attempt   Describe: _n/a_

      • Multiple Attempts   Describe: _n/a no attempts, only ideation_

(Y) N Current Intent   Describe: _feel must do something for pain_

Y **(N)** Impulsivity   Describe: _____

Y **(N)** Substance Abuse   Describe: _____

(Y) N Significant Loss   Describe: _obsessing over past girlfriend_

(Y) N Interpersonal Isolation   Describe: _feels he has cut himself off from others_

Y **(N)** Relationship Problems   Describe: _____

Y **(N)** Health Problems   Describe: _____

Y **(N)** Physical Pain   Describe: _____

Y **(N)** Legal Problems   Describe: _____

(Y) N Shame   Describe: _over father & family issues_

Section C (*Clinician*): OUTPATIENT TREATMENT PLAN (Refer to Sections A & B)

Problem #	Problem Description	Goals and Objectives Evidence for Attainment	Interventions (Type and Frequency)	Estimated # Sessions
1	*Self-Harm Potential*	*Outpatient Safety*	**Crisis Response Plan:** _Crisis Card avoid bridge read Choosing to Live_	_2x/wk for 4 weeks_
2	_unemployment_	_find a job_	_vocational assessment & counseling_	_4 weeks_
3	_social isolation_	_↑ social support_	_Problem solve to ↑ social support_	_4 weeks_

YES __✓__ NO _____ Patient understands and commits to outpatient treatment plan?

YES _____ NO __✓__ Clear and imminent danger of suicide?

_____   _____   _____   _____
Patient Signature   Date   Clinician Signature   Date

Section D (*Clinician Postsession Evaluation*):

MENTAL STATUS EXAM (circle appropriate items):

ALERTNESS: (ALERT) DROWSY LETHARGIC STUPOROUS
OTHER _____

ORIENTED TO: PERSON PLACE TIME REASON FOR EVALUATION x 4
MOOD: EUTHYMIC ELEVATED (DYSPHORIC) AGITATED ANGRY
AFFECT: FLAT BLUNTED CONSTRICTED APPROPRIATE (LABILE)
THOUGHT CONTINUITY: (CLEAR & COHERENT) GOAL-DIRECTED TANGENTIAL CIRCUMSTANTIAL
OTHER: _____

THOUGHT CONTENT: (WNL) OBSESSIONS DELUSIONS IDEAS OF REFERENCE BIZARRENESS MORBIDITY
OTHER: _____

ABSTRACTION: (WNL) NOTABLY CONCRETE
OTHER: _____

SPEECH: (WNL) RAPID SLOW SLURRED IMPOVERISHED INCOHERENT
OTHER: _____

MEMORY: (GROSSLY INTACT)
OTHER: _____

REALITY TESTING: (WNL) OTHER: _____

NOTABLE BEHAVIORAL OBSERVATIONS: *tearful, very upset* _____

PRELIMINARY DSM-IV-R MULTIAXIAL DIAGNOSES:

Axis I   *309.28 Adjust Dx & mixed anxiety/depressed mood*

Axis II   *defer*

Axis III   *n/a*

Axis IV   *prob. in social env./occupational issue*

Axis V   *50*

PATIENT'S OVERALL SUICIDE RISK LEVEL (check one and explain):

☐ No Significant Risk
☐ Mild
☒ Moderate
☐ Severe
☐ Extreme

Explanation: *Pt is depressed + anxious, has plan to jump,*
maybe use rifle, hx of S.I., but seems committed to 4tx,
open to Rx, no immediate danger, no need for hospitalization
at this time.

CASE NOTES (diagnosis, functional status, treatment plan, symptoms, prognosis, and progress to date):

Pt is a 24 y.o. white male, recent graduate who is unemployed. Socially isolating himself,
very depressed/anxious, tearful in session. But highly motivated to pursue outpatient 4tx and
possible Rx will refer to Dr. -. Will focus on intensive outpt. tx, monitor the suicidal ideation.

Next Appointment Scheduled: _____ Treatment Modality: *4tx + Rx consult*

_____   _____
Clinician Signature   Date   Supervisor Signature   Date

SSF-III SUICIDE TRACKING FORM

Patient: _____ Clinician: _____ Date: _____ Time: _____

Section A (*Patient*):

Rate each item according to how you feel <u>right now</u>.

1) **RATE PSYCHOLOGICAL PAIN** (*hurt, anguish, or misery in your mind; **not** stress; **not** physical pain*):

  Low Pain: 1 2 3 ④ 5 :High Pain

2) **RATE STRESS** (*your general feeling of being pressured or overwhelmed*):

  Low Stress: 1 2 3 ④ 5 :High Stress

3) **RATE AGITATION** (*emotional urgency; feeling that you need to take action; **not** irritation; **not** annoyance*):

  Low Agitation: 1 2 ③ 4 5 :High Agitation

4) **RATE HOPELESSNESS** (*your expectation that things will not get better no matter what you do*):

  Low Hopelessness: 1 2 3 ④ 5 :High Hopelessness

5) **RATE SELF-HATE** (*your general feeling of disliking yourself; having no self-esteem; having no self-respect*):

  Low Self-Hate: 1 2 3 ④ 5 :High Self-Hate

6) **RATE OVERALL RISK OF SUICIDE:**

  Extremely Low Risk: 1 ② 3 4 5 :Extremely High Risk
  (will <u>not</u> kill self)   (will kill self)

Section B (*Clinician*): Resolution of suicidality: ☐ 1st session ☐ 2nd session
Complete **SSF-III Suicide Tracking Outcome Form after third <u>consecutive</u> resolved session

Y ✓ N ___ Suicidal Thoughts?
Y ✓ N ___ Suicidal Feelings?
Y ___ N ✓ Suicidal Behaviors?

<u>Patient Status:</u>
☐ Discontinued treatment ☐ No show ☑ Referral to: *Dr. (Rx)* _____
☐ Hospitalization ☐ Cancelled ☐ Other: _____

TREATMENT PLAN UPDATE

Problem #	Problem Description	Goals and Objectives Evidence for Attainment	Interventions (Type and Frequency)	Estimated # Sessions
1	*Self-Harm Potential*	*Outpatient Safety*	**Crisis Response Plan:** *Crisis Card avoid bridge read book*	*2x/wk 4 weeks*
2	*depression + anxiety*	*↓depression ↓anxiety*	*CBT 4tx + Rx (Prozac)*	*4 weeks*
3	*unemployed*	*find a job*	*Behavioral plan to look for job*	*4 weeks*

_____   _____
Patient Signature   Date   Clinician Signature   Date

Section C *(Clinician Postsession Evaluation):*

MENTAL STATUS EXAM (circle appropriate items):

ALERTNESS: (ALERT) DROWSY LETHARGIC STUPOROUS
OTHER: _____

ORIENTED TO: PERSON PLACE TIME REASON FOR EVALUATION x 4

MOOD: EUTHYMIC ELEVATED (DYSPHORIC) AGITATED ANGRY *anxious*

AFFECT: FLAT BLUNTED CONSTRICTED APPROPRIATE LABILE

THOUGHT CONTINUITY: (CLEAR & COHERENT) GOAL-DIRECTED TANGENTIAL CIRCUMSTANTIAL
OTHER: _____

THOUGHT CONTENT: (WNL) OBSESSIONS DELUSIONS IDEAS OF REFERENCE BIZARRENESS MORBIDITY
OTHER: _____

ABSTRACTION: (WNL) NOTABLY CONCRETE
OTHER: _____

SPEECH: (WNL) RAPID SLOW SLURRED IMPOVERISHED INCOHERENT
OTHER: _____

MEMORY: (GROSSLY) INTACT
OTHER: _____

REALITY TESTING: (WNL) OTHER: _____

NOTABLE BEHAVIORAL OBSERVATIONS: *less tears in session*

DSM-IV-R MULTIAXIAL DIAGNOSES:

Axis I   309.28

Axis II   /

Axis III   /

Axis IV   *social/job issues*

Axis V   52

PATIENT'S OVERALL SUICIDE RISK LEVEL (check one and explain):

☐ No Significant Risk
☐ Mild
☒ Moderate
☐ Severe
☐ Extreme

Explanation: *Still has suicidal thoughts—but Crisis Card has worked—feels positive about taking Rx; very committed to tx plan. No imminent risk; no need for hospitalization*

CASE NOTES (diagnosis, functional status, treatment plan, symptoms, prognosis, and progress to date):

Pt somewhat composed, less emotional in session, open to be taking Rx. Used Crisis Card—positive experience—able to calm himself down, more stable, more able to focus on job hunt (developing structured beh. plan).

Next Appointment Scheduled: _____   Treatment Modality: *4tx + Rx*

_____   _____
Clinician Signature   Date   Supervisor Signature   Date

195

SSF-III SUICIDE TRACKING FORM

Patient: _____ Clinician: _____ Date: _____ Time: _____

Section A (*Patient*):

Rate each item according to how you feel <u>right now</u>.

1) **RATE PSYCHOLOGICAL PAIN** (*hurt, anguish, or misery in your mind;* **not** *stress;* **not** *physical pain*): Low Pain:　1　2　③　4　5　:High Pain
2) **RATE STRESS** (*your general feeling of being pressured or overwhelmed*): Low Stress:　1　2　3　④　5　:High Stress
3) **RATE AGITATION** (*emotional urgency; feeling that you need to take action;* **not** *irritation;* **not** *annoyance*): Low Agitation:　1　②　3　4　5　:High Agitation
4) **RATE HOPELESSNESS** (*your expectation that things will not get better no matter what you do*): Low Hopelessness:　1　2　3　④　5　:High Hopelessness
5) **RATE SELF-HATE** (*your general feeling of disliking yourself; having no self-esteem; having no self-respect*): Low Self-Hate:　1　2　3　④　5　:High Self-Hate
6) **RATE OVERALL RISK OF SUICIDE:** Extremely Low Risk:　1　②　3　4　5　:Extremely High Risk (will **not** kill self)　　　　　　　　　　　　　　　(will kill self)

Section B (*Clinician*):
Resolution of suicidality:　☐ 1st session　☐ 2nd session
Complete **SSF-III Suicide Tracking Outcome Form after third <u>consecutive</u> resolved session

Y ✓ N ___ Suicidal Thoughts?
Y ___ N ✓ Suicidal Feelings?
Y ___ N ✓ Suicidal Behaviors?

Patient Status:
☐ Discontinued treatment ☐ No show ☐ Referral to: _____
☐ Hospitalization ☐ Cancelled ☐ Other: _____

TREATMENT PLAN UPDATE

Problem #	Problem Description	Goals and Objectives Evidence for Attainment	Interventions (Type and Frequency)	Estimated # Sessions
1	Self-Harm Potential	Outpatient Safety	**Crisis Response Plan:** cont. Crisis Card	2x/wk 4 weeks
2	dep. + anx.	↓dep./anx.	CBJ + Rx	4 weeks
3	unemploy.	find job	beh. plan for job hunt	4 weeks

_____　　　　_____　　_____　　　　_____
Patient Signature　　　　　　　Date　　　　　Clinician Signature　　　　　　　Date

Section C (Clinician Postsession Evaluation):

MENTAL STATUS EXAM (circle appropriate items):

ALERTNESS: (ALERT) DROWSY LETHARGIC STUPOROUS
OTHER: _____

ORIENTED TO: PERSON PLACE TIME REASON FOR EVALUATION x 4

MOOD: EUTHYMIC ELEVATED DYSPHORIC AGITATED ANGRY *brighter*

AFFECT: FLAT BLUNTED CONSTRICTED (APPROPRIATE) LABILE

THOUGHT CONTINUITY: (CLEAR & COHERENT) GOAL-DIRECTED TANGENTIAL CIRCUMSTANTIAL
OTHER: _____

THOUGHT CONTENT: (WNL) OBSESSIONS DELUSIONS IDEAS OF REFERENCE BIZARRENESS MORBIDITY
OTHER: _____

ABSTRACTION: (WNL) NOTABLY CONCRETE
OTHER: _____

SPEECH: (WNL) RAPID SLOW SLURRED IMPOVERISHED INCOHERENT
OTHER: _____

MEMORY: (GROSSLY) INTACT
OTHER: _____

REALITY TESTING: (WNL) OTHER: _____

NOTABLE BEHAVIORAL OBSERVATIONS: *mood is better; no tears* _____

DSM-IV-R MULTIAXIAL DIAGNOSES:

Axis I _309.28_ _____

Axis II _/_ _____

Axis III _/_ _____

Axis IV _social/job_ _____

Axis V _55_ _____

PATIENT'S OVERALL SUICIDE RISK LEVEL (check one and explain):

☐ No Significant Risk
☐ Mild
☒ Moderate
☐ Severe
☐ Extreme

Explanation: *Still has some suicidal thoughts—but much less;*
using Crisis Card, very motivated for 4tx, no imminent risk
for suicide.

CASE NOTES (diagnosis, functional status, treatment plan, symptoms, prognosis, and progress to date):

Pt. is doing somewhat better—less tears, brighter affect. Pt. ↑ focus on job hunt + reaching out to others more. Has significant family of origin problems and history of neglect; abuse by father (who is depressed + alcoholic)

Next Appointment Scheduled: _____ Treatment Modality: _4tx + Rx_ _____

_____ _____

Clinician Signature   Date   Supervisor Signature   Date

SSF-III SUICIDE TRACKING FORM

Patient: _____ Clinician: _____ Date: _____ Time: _____

Section A (*Patient*):

Rate each item according to how you feel <u>right now</u>.

1) **RATE PSYCHOLOGICAL PAIN** (*hurt, anguish, or misery in your mind; **not** stress; **not** physical pain*):
Low Pain: 1 ② 3   4   5 :High Pain

2) **RATE STRESS** (*your general feeling of being pressured or overwhelmed*):
Low Stress: 1 ② 3   4   5 :High Stress

3) **RATE AGITATION** (*emotional urgency; feeling that you need to take action; **not** irritation; **not** annoyance*):
Low Agitation: 1 ② 3   4   5 :High Agitation

4) **RATE HOPELESSNESS** (*your expectation that things will not get better no matter what you do*):
Low Hopelessness: 1   2 ③ 4   5 :High Hopelessness

5) **RATE SELF-HATE** (*your general feeling of disliking yourself; having no self-esteem; having no self-respect*):
Low Self-Hate: 1   2 ③ 4   5 :High Self-Hate

6) **RATE OVERALL RISK OF SUICIDE:**
Extremely Low Risk: 1 ② 3   4   5 :Extremely High Risk (will <u>not</u> kill self)   (will kill self)

Section B (*Clinician*): Resolution of suicidality: ☐ 1st session ☐ 2nd session

Complete **SSF-III Suicide Tracking Outcome Form after third <u>consecutive</u> resolved session

Y ✓ N ___ Suicidal Thoughts? *"a little"*

Y ___ N ✓ Suicidal Feelings?

Y ___ N ✓ Suicidal Behaviors?

Patient Status:

☐ Discontinued treatment ☐ No show ☐ Referral to: _____

☐ Hospitalization ☐ Cancelled ☐ Other: _____

TREATMENT PLAN UPDATE

Problem #	Problem Description	Goals and Objectives Evidence for Attainment	Interventions (Type and Frequency)	Estimated # Sessions
1	*Self-Harm Potential*	*Outpatient Safety*	**Crisis Response Plan:** *Crisis Card*	*2x/wk 4 weeks*
2	*dep. + anx.*	*↓dep./anx.*	*CBT + Rx*	*4 weeks*
3	*unemploy.*	*find job + interview*	*beh. plan go on info interview*	*4 weeks*

_____   _____

Patient Signature   Date   Clinician Signature   Date

Section C *(Clinician Postsession Evaluation):*

MENTAL STATUS EXAM (circle appropriate items):

ALERTNESS: (ALERT) DROWSY LETHARGIC STUPOROUS
OTHER: _____

ORIENTED TO: PERSON PLACE TIME REASON FOR EVALUATION x 4

MOOD: EUTHYMIC ELEVATED DYSPHORIC AGITATED ANGRY

AFFECT: FLAT BLUNTED CONSTRICTED (APPROPRIATE) LABILE

THOUGHT CONTINUITY: (CLEAR & COHERENT) GOAL-DIRECTED TANGENTIAL CIRCUMSTANTIAL
OTHER: _____

THOUGHT CONTENT: (WNL) OBSESSIONS DELUSIONS IDEAS OF REFERENCE BIZARRENESS MORBIDITY
OTHER: _____

ABSTRACTION: (WNL) NOTABLY CONCRETE
OTHER: _____

SPEECH: (WNL) RAPID SLOW SLURRED IMPOVERISHED INCOHERENT
OTHER: _____

MEMORY: (GROSSLY) INTACT
OTHER: _____

REALITY TESTING: (WNL) OTHER: _____

NOTABLE BEHAVIORAL OBSERVATIONS: *doing better overall* _____

DSM-IV-R MULTIAXIAL DIAGNOSES:

Axis I _309.28_ _____

Axis II _/_ _____

Axis III _/_ _____

Axis IV _social/job_ _____

Axis V _58_ _____

PATIENT'S OVERALL SUICIDE RISK LEVEL (check one and explain):

☐ No Significant Risk   Explanation: _Still has some passive suicidal thoughts; but no plan &_
☑ Mild   _no imminent risk._
☐ Moderate
☐ Severe
☐ Extreme

CASE NOTES (diagnosis, functional status, treatment plan, symptoms, prognosis, and progress to date):

Pt. repeats feeling better; ↓ dep. ↓ anxiety—spending more time socially engaged, especially female
roommate. Pt. very focused on job search, will pursue info interview. Positive effect of Rx—feels
↑ energy ↑ focus.

Next Appointment Scheduled: _____ Treatment Modality: _4tx + Rx_ _____

_____   _____   _____   _____
Clinician Signature   Date   Supervisor Signature   Date

SSF-III SUICIDE TRACKING FORM

Patient: _____ Clinician: _____ Date: _____ Time: _____

Section A (*Patient*):

Rate each item according to how you feel right now.

1) **RATE PSYCHOLOGICAL PAIN** (*hurt, anguish, or misery in your mind; **not** stress; **not** physical pain*):   Low Pain: 1 ② 3 4 5 :High Pain
2) **RATE STRESS** (*your general feeling of being pressured or overwhelmed*):   Low Stress: 1 ② 3 4 5 :High Stress
3) **RATE AGITATION** (*emotional urgency; feeling that you need to take action; **not** irritation; **not** annoyance*):   Low Agitation: ① 2 3 4 5 :High Agitation
4) **RATE HOPELESSNESS** (*your expectation that things will not get better no matter what you do*):   Low Hopelessness: 1 ② 3 4 5 :High Hopelessness
5) **RATE SELF-HATE** (*your general feeling of disliking yourself; having no self-esteem; having no self-respect*):   Low Self-Hate: 1 ② 3 4 5 :High Self-Hate

6) **RATE OVERALL RISK OF SUICIDE:**
  Extremely Low Risk: ① 2 3 4 5 :Extremely High Risk
  (will **not** kill self)   (will kill self)

Section B (*Clinician*): | Resolution of suicidality: ☑ 1st session ☐ 2nd session
Complete **SSF-III Suicide Tracking Outcome Form after third <u>consecutive</u> resolved session

Y ___ N ✓ Suicidal Thoughts?
Y ___ N ✓ Suicidal Feelings?
Y ___ N ✓ Suicidal Behaviors?

Patient Status:
☐ Discontinued treatment ☐ No show ☐ Referral to: _____
☐ Hospitalization   ☐ Cancelled ☐ Other: _____

TREATMENT PLAN UPDATE

Problem #	Problem Description	Goals and Objectives Evidence for Attainment	Interventions (Type and Frequency)	Estimated # Sessions
1	Self-Harm Potential	Outpatient Safety	**Crisis Response Plan:** Crisis Card	2x/wk
2	dep. + anx.	↓dep./anx.	CBT + Rx	4 weeks
3	job issues	find job	beh. plan— Pt. will seek info interviews	4 weeks

_____   _____   _____   _____
Patient Signature   Date   Clinician Signature   Date

Section C (Clinician Postsession Evaluation):

MENTAL STATUS EXAM (circle appropriate items):

ALERTNESS: (ALERT) DROWSY LETHARGIC STUPOROUS
OTHER: _____

ORIENTED TO: PERSON PLACE TIME REASON FOR EVALUATION x 4

MOOD: EUTHYMIC ELEVATED DYSPHORIC AGITATED ANGRY

AFFECT: FLAT BLUNTED CONSTRICTED (APPROPRIATE) LABILE

THOUGHT CONTINUITY: (CLEAR & COHERENT) GOAL-DIRECTED TANGENTIAL CIRCUMSTANTIAL
OTHER: _____

THOUGHT CONTENT: (WNL) OBSESSIONS DELUSIONS IDEAS OF REFERENCE BIZARRENESS MORBIDITY
OTHER: _____

ABSTRACTION: (WNL) NOTABLY CONCRETE
OTHER: _____

SPEECH: (WNL) RAPID SLOW SLURRED IMPOVERISHED INCOHERENT
OTHER: _____

MEMORY: (GROSSLY) INTACT
OTHER: _____

REALITY TESTING: (WNL) OTHER: _____

NOTABLE BEHAVIORAL OBSERVATIONS: _doing well; no suicidal thoughts_ _____

DSM-IV-R MULTIAXIAL DIAGNOSES:

Axis I _309.28_ _____

Axis II _/_ _____

Axis III _/_ _____

Axis IV _social/job_ _____

Axis V _63_ _____

PATIENT'S OVERALL SUICIDE RISK LEVEL (check one and explain):

☐ No Significant Risk   Explanation: _says suicidal ideation gone; not even passing thoughts—_
☑ Mild   _no intent, no apparent suicidal risk_ _____
☐ Moderate _____
☐ Severe _____
☐ Extreme _____

CASE NOTES (diagnosis, functional status, treatment plan, symptoms, prognosis, and progress to date):

Pt. cont. to improve; rel. + roommate very helpful. Feeling more patient about job hunt. ↑energy
↑ soc. support; Rx seems to be helping. Cont. to discuss family issues.

Next Appointment Scheduled: _____   Treatment Modality: _4tx + Rx_ _____

Clinician Signature   Date   Supervisor Signature   Date

SSF-III SUICIDE TRACKING FORM

Patient: _____ Clinician: _____ Date: _____ Time: _____

Section A (*Patient*):

Rate each item according to how you feel <u>right now</u>.

| 1) **RATE PSYCHOLOGICAL PAIN** (*hurt, anguish, or misery in your mind; **not** stress; **not** physical pain*): |
| Low Pain: 1   2   ③   4   5   :High Pain |

| 2) **RATE STRESS** (*your general feeling of being pressured or overwhelmed*): |
| Low Stress: 1   2   ③   4   5   :High Stress |

| 3) **RATE AGITATION** (*emotional urgency; feeling that you need to take action; **not** irritation; **not** annoyance*): |
| Low Agitation: 1   2   ③   4   5   :High Agitation |

| 4) **RATE HOPELESSNESS** (*your expectation that things will not get better no matter what you do*): |
| Low Hopelessness: 1   ②   3   4   5   :High Hopelessness |

| 5) **RATE SELF-HATE** (*your general feeling of disliking yourself; having no self-esteem; having no self-respect*): |
| Low Self-Hate: 1   2   ③   4   5   :High Self-Hate |

| 6) **RATE OVERALL RISK OF SUICIDE:** |
| Extremely Low Risk: ①   2   3   4   5   :Extremely High Risk
 (will <u>not</u> kill self)   (will kill self) |

Section B (*Clinician*):   Resolution of suicidality: ☐ 1st session   ☑ 2nd session
                  Complete SSF-III Suicide Tracking Outcome Form after third <u>consecutive</u> resolved session

Y ___ N ✓ Suicidal Thoughts?   <u>Patient Status:</u>
Y ___ N ✓ Suicidal Feelings?   ☐ Discontinued treatment ☐ No show   ☐ Referral to: _____
Y ___ N ✓ Suicidal Behaviors?   ☐ Hospitalization   ☐ Cancelled   ☐ Other: _____

TREATMENT PLAN UPDATE

Problem #	Problem Description	Goals and Objectives Evidence for Attainment	Interventions (Type and Frequency)	Estimated # Sessions
1	*Self-Harm Potential*	*Outpatient Safety*	**Crisis Response Plan:** *Cont. Crisis Card seek soc. support*	*2x/wk*
2	*dep. + anx.*	*↓ dep./anx.*	*CBT + Rx*	*4 weeks*
3	*relationship crisis*	*resolve crisis in new relationship*	*problem solve possible couples tx?*	*4 weeks*

_____   _____   _____   _____
Patient Signature   Date   Clinician Signature   Date

Section C *(Clinician Postsession Evaluation):*

MENTAL STATUS EXAM (circle appropriate items):

ALERTNESS: (ALERT) DROWSY LETHARGIC STUPOROUS
OTHER: _____

ORIENTED TO: PERSON PLACE TIME REASON FOR EVALUATION × 4

MOOD: EUTHYMIC ELEVATED DYSPHORIC (AGITATED) ANGRY

AFFECT: FLAT BLUNTED CONSTRICTED (APPROPRIATE) LABILE

THOUGHT CONTINUITY: (CLEAR & COHERENT) GOAL-DIRECTED TANGENTIAL CIRCUMSTANTIAL
OTHER: _____

THOUGHT CONTENT: (WNL) OBSESSIONS DELUSIONS IDEAS OF REFERENCE BIZARRENESS MORBIDITY
OTHER: _____

ABSTRACTION: (WNL) NOTABLY CONCRETE
OTHER: _____

SPEECH: (WNL) RAPID SLOW SLURRED IMPOVERISHED INCOHERENT
OTHER: _____

MEMORY: (GROSSLY) INTACT
OTHER: _____

REALITY TESTING: (WNL) OTHER: _____

NOTABLE BEHAVIORAL OBSERVATIONS: *Pt. upset w/self over fight w/female friend*

DSM-IV-R MULTIAXIAL DIAGNOSES:

Axis I _____309.28_____

Axis II _____/_____

Axis III _____/_____

Axis IV _____social/job_____

Axis V _____61_____

PATIENT'S OVERALL SUICIDE RISK LEVEL (check one and explain):

☑ No Significant Risk   Explanation: *Pt. had 1 episode of a "flash" of suicidal thought during*
☐ Mild
☐ Moderate   *fight w/female friend—used Crisis Card and calmed down; insists that*
☐ Severe   *suicide is not an option*
☐ Extreme

CASE NOTES (diagnosis, functional status, treatment plan, symptoms, prognosis, and progress to date):

Pt. has been doing very well—has gotten romantically involved w/roommate. They got into fight
over past girlfriend of pt. Had "flash" of suicidal ideation during fight, but quickly recovered.
They are talking, trying to work things out; asked about couples tx?

Next Appointment Scheduled: _____ Treatment Modality: *4tx + Rx*

_____   _____
Clinician Signature   Date   Supervisor Signature   Date

SSF-III SUICIDE TRACKING OUTCOME FORM

Patient: _____ Clinician: _____ Date: _____ Time: _____

Section A (*Patient*):

Rate each item according to how you feel <u>right now</u>.

1) **RATE PSYCHOLOGICAL PAIN** (*hurt, anguish, or misery in your mind; **not** stress; **not** physical pain*): Low Pain: (①) 2   3   4   5   :High Pain
2) **RATE STRESS** (*your general feeling of being pressured or overwhelmed*): Low Stress: (①) 2   3   4   5   :High Stress
3) **RATE AGITATION** (*emotional urgency; feeling that you need to take action; **not** irritation; **not** annoyance*): Low Agitation: (①) 2   3   4   5   :High Agitation
4) **RATE HOPELESSNESS** (*your expectation that things will not get better no matter what you do*): Low Hopelessness: (①) 2   3   4   5   :High Hopelessness
5) **RATE SELF-HATE** (*your general feeling of disliking yourself; having no self-esteem; having no self-respect*): Low Self-Hate: (①) 2   3   4   5   :High Self-Hate
6) **RATE OVERALL RISK OF SUICIDE:** Extremely Low Risk: (①) 2   3   4   5   :Extremely High Risk (will <u>not</u> kill self)   (will kill self)

Were there any aspects of your treatment that were particularly helpful to you? If so, please describe these. Be as specific as possible.

Combination of medicine and counseling

Getting perspective on job search

_____

What have you learned from your clinical care that could help you if you became suicidal in the future?

Crisis Card worked! Journaling really helps too.

I have learned to seek support from friends.

_____

Section B (*Clinician*):

Third consecutive session of resolved suicidality: Yes ✓ No ____ (if No, continue Suicide Status Tracking)

<u>**OUTCOME/DISPOSITION**</u> (Check all that apply):

✓ Continuing outpatient psychotherapy ____ Inpatient hospitalization

____ Mutual termination ____ Patient chooses to discontinued treatment (unilaterally)

____ Referral to: _____

____ Other. Describe: _____

Next Appointment Scheduled (if applicable): *we will consider 1x/wk if pt. remains stable*

_____   _____
Patient Signature   Date   Clinician Signature   Date

Section C (*Clinician Outcome Evaluation*)

MENTAL STATUS EXAM (circle appropriate items):

ALERTNESS: (ALERT) DROWSY LETHARGIC STUPOROUS
OTHER: _____

ORIENTED TO: PERSON PLACE TIME REASON FOR EVALUATION $\times$ 4

MOOD: EUTHYMIC ELEVATED DYSPHORIC AGITATED ANGRY

AFFECT: FLAT BLUNTED CONSTRICTED (APPROPRIATE) LABILE

THOUGHT CONTINUITY: (CLEAR & COHERENT) GOAL-DIRECTED TANGENTIAL CIRCUMSTANTIAL
OTHER: _____

THOUGHT CONTENT: (WNL) OBSESSIONS DELUSIONS IDEAS OF REFERENCE BIZARRENESS MORBIDITY
OTHER: _____

ABSTRACTION: (WNL) NOTABLY CONCRETE
OTHER: _____

SPEECH: (WNL) RAPID SLOW SLURRED IMPOVERISHED INCOHERENT
OTHER: _____

MEMORY: (GROSSLY) INTACT
OTHER: _____

REALITY TESTING: (WNL) OTHER: _____

NOTABLE BEHAVIORAL OBSERVATIONS: *Pt. doing very well - happy w/positive attitude*

DSM-IV-R MULTIAXIAL DIAGNOSES:

Axis I   _309.28_

Axis II   _/_

Axis III _/_

Axis IV   _/_

Axis V   _70_

PATIENT'S OVERALL SUICIDE RISK LEVEL (check one and explain):

☑ No Significant Risk   Explanation: *Pt. has completely resolved suicidality: "no longer an*
☐ Mild   *option for me."*
☐ Moderate   _____
☐ Severe   _____
☐ Extreme

CASE NOTES (diagnosis, functional status, treatment plan, symptoms, prognosis, and progress to date):

Pt. has progressed very well. Suicidal ideation is completely extinguished. Pt. is pursuing job in
systematic way. Feeling positive about getting good job. Pt. is in new relationship that is very
positive; Pt.↑ socially involved. Wants to continue 4tx/Rx w/↑ focus on family of origin,
particularly issues w/father.

Next Appointment Scheduled: _____   Treatment Modality: *4tx + Rx*

_____   _____
Clinician Signature   Date   Supervisor Signature   Date

References

Adler, G., & Buie, D. H., Jr. (1979). Aloneness and borderline psychopathology: The possible relevance of child development issues. *International Journal of Psychoanalysis, 60,* 83–96.

American Psychiatric Association. (1994). *Diagnostic and statistical manual of mental disorders* (4th ed.). Washington, DC: Author.

Bakan, D. (1966). *The duality of human existence.* Chicago: Rand McNally.

Baumeister, R. F. (1990). Suicide as escape from self. *Psychological Review, 97,* 90–113.

Beck, A. T. (1967). *Depression: Clinical, experimental, and theoretical aspects.* New York: Harper & Row.

Beck, A. T. (1986). Hopelessness as a predictor of eventual suicide. *Annals of New York Academy of Sciences, 487,* 90–96.

Beck, A. T., & Steer, R. A. (1988). *Manual for the Beck Hopelessness Scale.* San Antonio, TX: Psychological Corporation.

Beck, A. T., Rush, A. J., Shaw, B. F., & Emery, G. (1979). *Cognitive therapy of depression.* New York: Guilford Press.

Beck, A. T., Steer, R. A., Kovacs, M., & Garrison, B. (1985). Hopelessness and eventual suicide: A 10-year prospective study of patients hospitalized with suicidal ideation. *American Journal of Psychiatry, 142,* 559–563.

Berman, A. L., & Jobes, D. A. (1991). *Adolescent suicide: Assessment and intervention.* Washington, DC: American Psychological Association.

Berman, A. L., Jobes, D. A., & Silverman, M. M. (2006). *Adolescent suicide: Assessment and intervention* (2nd ed.). Washington, DC: American Psychological Association.

Brown, G. K., Beck, A. T., Steer, R. A., & Grisham, J. R. (2000). Risk factors for suicide in psychiatric outpatients: A 20-year prospective study. *Journal of Consulting and Clinical Psychology, 68,* 371–377.

Brown, G. K., Have, T. T., Henriques, G. R., Xie, S. X., Hollander, J. E., & Beck, A. T. (2005)

Cognitive therapy for the prevention of suicide attempts. *Journal of the American Medical Association, 294,* 563–570.

Brown, G. K., Steer, R. A., Henriques, G. R., & Beck, A. T. (2005). The internal struggle between the wish to die and the wish to live: A risk factor for suicide. *American Journal of Psychiatry, 162,* 1977–1979.

Chiles, J. A., & Strosahl, K. D. (1995). *The suicidal patient: Principles of assessment, treatment, and case management.* Washington, DC: American Psychiatric Association.

Comtois, K. A., Jobes, D. A., & Morgan, A. (2005). *Collaborative assessment and management of suicide for next day appointments for suicidal patients.* Unpublished research grant proposal.

Coombs, D. W., Miller, H. L., Alarcon, R., Herlihy, C., Lee, J. M., & Morrison, D. P. (1992). Presuicide attempt communications between parasuicides and consulted caregivers. *Suicide and Life-Threatening Behavior, 22,* 289–302.

Crumlish, J. A. (1996). *Therapist responses to difficult patient presentations.* Unpublished doctoral dissertation, The Catholic University of America, Washington, DC.

Derogatis, L. R., Lipman, R. S., Rickels, K., Uhlenhuth, E. H., & Covi, L. (1974). The Hopkins Symptom Checklist (HSCL): A self-report symptom inventory. *Behavioral Science, 19,* 1–15.

Derogatis, L. R., Rickels, K., & Rock, A. (1976). The SCL-90 and the MMPI: A step in the validation of a new self-report scale. *British Journal of Psychiatry, 128,* 280–289.

Derogatis, L. R., & Savitz, K. L. (1999). The SCL-90-R, Brief Symptom Inventory, and Matching Clinical Rating Scales. In M. E. Maruish (Ed.), *The use of psychological testing for treatment planning and outcomes assessment.* Mahwah, NJ: Erlbaum.

Drozd, J. F., Jobes, D. A., & Luoma, J. B. (2000). The collaborative assessment and management of suicidality in air force mental health clinics. *The Air Force Psychologist, 18,* 6–11.

Eddins, C. L., & Jobes, D. A. (1994). Do you see what I see? Patient and clinician perceptions of underlying dimensions of suicidality. *Suicide and Life-Threatening Behavior, 24,* 170–173.

Elkin, I., Shea, M., Watkins, J. T., Imber, S. D., Sotsky, S. M., Collins, J. F., et al. (1989). National Institute of Mental Health Treatment of Depression Collaborative Research Program: General effectiveness of treatments. *Archives of General Psychiatry, 46,* 971–982.

Ellis, T. E. (2004). Collaboration and a self-help orientation in therapy with suicidal clients. *Journal of Contemporary Psychotherapy, 34,* 41–57.

Ellis, T. E., & Newman, C. F. (1996). *Choosing to live: How to defeat suicide through cognitive therapy.* Oakland, CA: New Harbinger.

Fazaa, N., & Page, S. (2003). Dependency and self-criticism as predictors of suicidal behavior. *Suicide and Life-Threatening Behavior, 33,* 172–185.

Fazaa, N., & Page, S. (2005). Two distinct personality configurations: Understanding the therapeutic context with suicidal individuals. *Journal of Contemporary Psychotherapy, 35,* 331–346.

Figueroa, R., Harman, J., & Engberg, J. (2004). Use of claims data to examine the impact of length of inpatient psychiatric stay on readmission rate. *Psychiatric Services, 55,* 560–565.

Fratto, T., Jobes, D. A., Pentiuc, D., Rice, R., & Tendick, V. (2004). *The SSF One-Thing Assessment for Suicidal Risk.* Unpublished manuscript, The Catholic University of America, Washington, DC.

Garfield, S. L. (1994). Research on client variables in psychotherapy. In A. E. Bergin & S. L. Garfield (Eds.), *Handbook of psychotherapy and behavior change* (4th ed., pp. 190–228). New York: Wiley.

Gay, P. (1989). *The Freud reader.* New York: Norton.

Goldstein, J. (1993). Psychiatry. In W. F. Bynum & R. Porter (Eds.), *Companion encyclopedia of the history of medicine* (Vol. 2, pp. 1350–1372). New York: Routledge.

Hendin, H., Haas, A. P., Maltsberger, J. T., Szanto, K., & Rabinowicz, H. (2004). Factors contributing to therapists' distress after the suicide of a patient. *American Journal of Psychiatry, 161,* 1442–1446.

Henriques, G., Beck, A. T., & Brown, G. K. (2003). Cognitive therapy for adolescent and young adult suicide attempters. *American Behavioral Scientist, 46,* 1258–1268.

Horvath, A. O., & Symonds, B. D. (1991). Relationship between working alliance and outcome in psychotherapy: A meta-analyisis. *Journal of Counseling Psychology, 38,* 139–149.

Jacoby, A. M. (2003). *Negative countertransference in psychotherapy with suicidal patients.* Unpublished doctoral dissertation, The Catholic University of America, Washington, DC.

Jacobson, N. S., Martell, C. R., & Dimidjian, S. (2001). Behavioral activation treatment for depression. *Clinical Psychology: Science and Practice, 8,* 255–270.

Jobes, D. A. (1995a). The challenge and promise of clinical suicidology. *Suicide and Life-Threatening Behavior, 25,* 437–449.

Jobes, D. A. (1995b). Psychodynamic treatment of adolescent suicide attempters. In J. Zimmerman & G. M. Asnis (Eds.), *Treatment approaches with suicidal adolescents* (pp. 137–154). New York: Wiley.

Jobes, D. A. (2000). Collaborating to prevent suicide: A clinical-research perspective. *Suicide and Life-Threatening Behavior, 30,* 8–17.

Jobes, D. A. (2001, April). *Quantitative/qualitative assessment of suicidality.* Paper presented at the annual meeting of the American Association of Suicidology, Atlanta, GA.

Jobes, D. A. (2003). Understanding suicide in the 21st century. *Preventing Suicide: The National Journal, 2,* 2–4.

Jobes, D. A. (2004a, April). *Crisis center use of the SSF.* Workshop presentation at the annual conference of the American Association of Suicidology, Miami, FL.

Jobes, D. A. (2004b, October). *The psychology of suicide: Research on what suicidal patients have to say.* Keynote address at the 3rd annual Military Suicide Prevention Conference, Crystal City, VA.

Jobes, D. A. (2005). *Assessing and treating suicidal college students.* Unpublished research grant proposal.

Jobes, D. A., & Berman, A. L. (1993). Suicide and malpractice liability: Assessing and revising policies, procedures, and practice in outpatient settings. *Professional Psychology: Research and Practice, 24,* 91 99.

Jobes, D. A., & Bostwick, J. M. (2006, April). *Perturbed suicidality: Research and treatment.* Research presentation at the annual conference of the American Association of Suicidology, Seattle, WA.

Jobes, D. A., Casey, J. O., Berman, A. L., & Wright, D. G. (1991). Empirical criteria for the determination of suicide manner of death. *Journal of Forensic Sciences, 36,* 244–256.

Jobes, D. A., & Drozd, J. F. (2004). The CAMS approach to working with suicidal patients. *Journal of Contemporary Psychotherapy, 34,* 73–85.

Jobes, D. A., Eyman, J. R., & Yufit, R. I. (1995). How clinicians assess suicide risk in adolescents and adults. *Crisis Intervention and Time-Limited Treatment, 2,* 1–12.

Jobes, D. A., & Flemming, E. P. (2004, August). *Qualitative SSF assessments of suicidality and treatment outcome.* Paper presented at the 10th European Symposium on Suicide and Suicide Behaviors, Copenhagen, Denmark.

Jobes, D. A., Jacoby, A. M., Cimbolic, P., & Hustead, L. A. T. (1997). Assessment and treatment of suicidal clients in a university counseling center. *Journal of Counseling Psychology, 44,* 368–377.

Jobes, D. A., & Karmel, M. P. (1996). Case consultation with a suicidal adolescent. In A. Leenaars & D. Lester (Eds.), *Suicide and the unconscious* (pp. 175–193). Northvale, NJ: Aronson.

Jobes, D. A., Luoma, J. B., Jacoby, A. M., & Mann, R. E. (1998). *Manual for the collaborative assessment and management of suicidality (CAMS).* Unpublished manuscript, The Catholic University of America, Washington, DC.

Jobes, D. A., & Maltsberger, J. T. (1995). The hazards of treating suicidal patients. In M. B. Sussman (Ed.), *A perilous calling: The hazards of psychotherapy practice* (pp. 200–214). New York: Wiley.

Jobes, D. A., & Mann, R. E. (1999). Reasons for living versus reasons for dying: Examining the internal debate of suicide. *Suicide and Life-Threatening Behavior, 29,* 97–104.

Jobes, D. A., & Mann, R. E. (2000). Letters to the editor—Reply. *Suicide and Life-Threatening Behavior, 30,* 182.

Jobes, D. A., & Nelson, K. N. (2006). Shneidman's contributions to the understanding of suicidal thinking. In T. E. Ellis (Ed.), *Cognition and suicide: Theory, research, and therapy* (pp. 29–49). Washington, DC: American Psychological Association.

Jobes, D. A., Nelson, K. N., Peterson, E. M., Pentiuc, D., Downing, V., Francini, K., et al. (2004). Describing suicidality: An investigation of qualitative SSF responses. *Suicide and Life-Threatening Behavior, 34,* 99–112.

Jobes, D. A., Wong, S. A., Conrad, A., Drozd, J. F., & Neal-Walden, T. (2005). The Collaborative assessment and management of suicidality vs. treatment as usual: A retrospective study with suicidal outpatients. *Suicide and Life-Threatening Behavior, 35,* 483–497.

Joiner, T. E. (2005). *Why people die by suicide.* Boston: Harvard University Press.

Joiner, T. E., Conwell, Y., Fitzpatrick, K. K., Witte, T. K., Schmidt, N. B., Berlim, M. T., et al. (2005). Four studies on how past and current suicidality relate even when "everything but the kitchen sink" is covaried. *Journal of Abnormal Psychology, 114,* 291–303.

Joiner, T. E., Walker, R. L., Rudd, M. D., & Jobes, D. A. (1999). Scientizing and routinizing the assessment of suicidality in outpatient practice. *Professional Psychology: Research and Practice, 30*, 447–453.

Judd, S., Jobes, D. A., Arnkoff, D. B., & Fenton, W. (1999). *Negative countertransference and suicide: An empirical evaluation.* Unpublished manuscript, The Catholic University of America, Washington, DC.

Kahn-Greene, E. T., Jobes, D. A., Goeke-Morey, M., & Green, J. (2006). *Trajectories of improvement in suicidal individuals: Examining Suicide Status Form responses as moderators.* Unpublished manuscript, The Catholic University of America, Washington, DC.

Kopta, S. M., & Lowry, J. L. (2002). Psychometric Evaluation of the Behavioral Health Questionnaire–20: A brief instrument for assessing global mental health and the three phases of psychotherapy outcome. *Society for Psychotherapy Research, 12*, 413–426.

Kovacs, M., & Beck, A. T. (1977). The wish to die and the wish to live in attempted suicides. *Journal of Clinical Psychology, 33*, 361–365.

Lambert, M. J., Hansen, N. B, Umphress, V., Lunnen, K., Okiishi, J., Burlingame, G., et al. (1996). *Administration and scoring manual for the Outcome Questionnaire (OQ 45.2).* Wilmington, DE: American Professional Credentialing Services.

Lambert, M. J., Burlingame, G., Umphress, V., Hansen, N., Vermeersch, D., Clouse, G., et al. (1996). The reliability and validity of the Outcome Questionnaire. *Clinical Psychology and Psychotherapy, 3*, 106–116.

Leenaars, A. A. (2004). *Psychotherapy with suicidal people: A person-centered approach.* New York: Wiley.

Lineberry, T. W., Brancu, M., Varghese, R., Jobes, D. A., Jacoby, A. M., Conrad, A. K., et al. (2006, March). *Clinical use of the suicide status form on a psychiatric inpatient unit.* Poster presented at the Fourth Aeschi Conference, Aeschi, Switzerland.

Linehan, M. M. (1993a). *Cognitive-behavioral treatment of borderline personality disorder.* New York: Guilford Press.

Linehan, M. M. (1993b). *Skills training manual for treating borderline personality disorder.* New York: Guilford Press.

Linehan, M. M. (1998, April). *Is anything effective for reducing suicidal behavior?* Paper presented at the annual meeting of the American Association of Suicidology, Bethesda, MD.

Linehan, M. M. (2005, August). *Latest research on suicide and DBT.* Paper presented at the annual convention of the American Psychological Association, Washington, DC.

Linehan, M. M., Armstrong, H. E., Suarez, A., Allmon, D., & Heard, H. L. (1991). Cognitive-behavioral treatment of chronically parasuicidal borderline patients. *Archives of General Psychiatry, 48*, 1060–1064.

Linehan, M. M., Goodstein, J. L., Nielsen, S. L., & Chiles, J. A. (1983). Reasons for staying alive when you are thinking of killing yourself: The reasons for living inventory. *Journal of Consulting and Clinical Psychology, 51*, 276–286.

Luoma, J. B. (1999). *Student's perceptions of items on the suicide status form.* Unpublished manuscript, The Catholic University of American, Washington, DC.

Luoma, J. B., Martin, K. E., & Pearson, J. L. (2002). Contact with mental health and primary care providers before suicide: A review of the evidence. *American Journal of Psychiatry, 159*, 909–916.

Maltsberger, J. T. (1994). Calculated risk-taking in the treatment of suicidal patients: Ethical and legal problems. In A. Leenaars, J. Maltsberger, & R. Neimeyer (Eds.), Treatment of suicidal people (pp. 195–205). Washington, DC: Taylor & Francis.

Maltsberger, J. T., & Buie, E. H. (1974). Countertransference hate in the treatment of suicidal patients. *Archives of General Psychiatry, 30,* 625–633.

Mann, R. (2002). *Reasons for living vs. reasons for dying: The development of suicidal typologies for predicting treatment outcomes.* Unpublished dissertation, The Catholic University of America, Washington, DC.

Maris, R. W., Berman, A, L., & Silverman, M. M. (2000). *Comprehensive textbook of suicidology.* New York: Guilford Press.

Michel, K., Maltsberger, J. T., Jobes, D. A., Leenaars, A., Orbach, I., Young, R., et al. (2002). Discovering the truth in attempted suicide. *American Journal of Psychotherapy, 56,* 424–437.

Michel, K., Valach, L., & Waeber, V. (1994). Understanding deliberate self-harm: The patient's view. *Crisis, 15,* 172–178.

Millon, T. (2004). *Masters of the mind: Exploring the story of mental illness from ancient times to the new millennium.* Hoboken, NJ: Wiley.

Mishara, B. L., Chagnon, F., Daigle, M., Bogdan, B., Raymond, S., Marcous, I., et al. (2005, April). *Practical implications for crisis centers of the AAS-Hopeline Silent Monitoring Evaluation Study.* Paper presented at the annual conference of the American Association of Suicidology, Denver, CO.

Motto, J. A. (1976). Suicide prevention for high-risk persons who refuse treatment. *Suicide and Life-Threatening Behavior, 6,* 223–230.

Motto, J. A., & Bostrom, A. G. (2001). A randomized controlled trial of postcrisis suicide prevention. *Psychiatric Services, 52,* 828–833.

Murray, H. A. (1938). *Explorations in personality.* New York: Oxford University Press.

Nademin, E., Jobes, D. A., Downing, V. & Mann, R. (2005). *Reasons for living among college students: A comparison between suicidal and non-suicidal samples.* Unpublished manuscript, The Catholic University of America, Washington, DC.

National Alliance for the Mentally Ill. (2000, November 17). *Outpatient services experience big decline in availability according to new study* (Press release). Available at www.nami.org.

O'Connor, R. C., O'Connor, D. B., O'Connor, S. M., Smallwood, J., & Miles, J. (2004). Hopelessness, stress, perfectionism: The moderating effects of future thinking. *Cognitions and Emotions, 18,* 1099–1120.

Olfson, M., Gameroff, M. J., Marcus, S. C., Greenberg, T., & Shaffer, D. (2005). National trends in hospitalization of youth with intentional self-inflicted injuries. *American Journal of Psychiatry, 162,* 1328–1335.

Oordt, M., Jobes, D., Rudd, M., Fonseca, V., Russ, C., Stea, J., et al. (2005). Development of a clinical guide to enhance care for suicidal patients. *Professional Psychology: Research and Practice, 36,* 208–218.

Oordt, M., Fonseca, V. P., Schmidt, S. M, & Jobes, D. A. (2005). *Educating mental health professionals to assess and manage suicidal behavior: Can provider confidence and practice behaviors be altered?* Manuscript submitted for publication.

Orbach, I. (2001). Therapeutic empathy with the suicidal wish. *American Journal of Psychotherapy, 55*, 166–184.

Overholser, J. C. (2005). Contemporary psychotherapy: Promoting personal responsibility for therapeutic change. *Journal of Contemporary Psychotherapy, 35*, 369–376.

Peterson, E. M. (2003). *Assessing suicide risk and predicting treatment outcomes: The role of suicide history, suicide status form qualitative responses, and response style.* Unpublished doctoral dissertation, The Catholic University of America, Washington, DC.

Peterson, E. M., Luoma, J. B., & Dunne, E. (2002). Suicide survivors' perceptions of the treating clinician. *Suicide and Life-Threatening Behavior, 32*, 158–166.

Pope, K. S., & Tabachnik, B. G. (1993). Therapists' anger, fear, and sexual feelings: National survey of therapist responses, client characteristics, critical, formal complaints, and training. *Professional Psychology: Research and Practice, 24*, 142–152.

Range, L. M., & Penton, S. R. (1994). Hope, hopelessness, and suicidality in college students. *Psychological Reports, 75*, 456–458.

Rice, R. E. (2002). *Assessing agentic and communal traits in suicidal outpatients: A potential model for predicting typologies, severity, and treatment outcome.* Unpublished doctoral dissertation, The Catholic University of America, Washington, DC.

Rotter, J. B., & Rafferty, J. E. (1950). *Manual for the Rotter Incomplete Sentence Blank, college form.* New York: Psychological Corporation.

Rudd, M., & Joiner, T. (1998). Relationships among suicide ideators, attempters, and multiples attempters in a young adult sample. *Journal of Abnormal Psychology, 105*, 541–550.

Rudd, M. D., Joiner, T., Jobes, D. A., & King, C. A. (1999). Practice guidelines in the outpatient treatment of suicidality: An integration of science and a recognition of its limitations. *Professional Psychology: Research and Practice, 30*, 437–446.

Rudd, M.D., Joiner, T., & Rajab, M. H. (2001). *Treating suicidal behavior: An effective, time-limited approach.* New York: Guilford Press.

Rudd, M. D., Mandrusiak, M., & Joiner, T. (2006). The case against no-suicide contracts: The commitment to treatment statement as a practice alternative. *Journal of Clinical Psychology, 62*, 243–251.

Shea, S. C. (1999). *The practical art of suicide assessment: A guide for mental health professionals and substance abuse counselors.* New York: Wiley.

Schilling, N., Harbauer, G., Andreae, A., & Haas, S. (2006, March). *Suicide risk assessment in inpatient crisis intervention.* Poster presented at the Fourth Aeschi Conference, Aeschi, Switzerland.

Shneidman, E. S. (1985). *The definition of suicide.* New York: Wiley.

Shneidman, E. S. (1987). A psychological approach to suicide. In G. R. Vanden Box & B. K. Bryant (Eds.), *Cataclysms, crises, and catastrophies: Psychology in action* (pp. 147–183). Washington, DC: American Psychological Association.

Shneidman, E. S. (1988). Some reflections of a founder. *Suicide and Life-Threatening Behavior, 18*, 1–12.

Shneidman, E. (1993). *Suicide as psychache: A clinical approach to self-destructive behavior.* Northvale, NJ: Aronson.

Shneidman, E. S. (1998). *The suicidal mind.* Northfield, NJ: Jason Aronson.

Weinstein, M. J. (2002). *Psychotherapy progress of suicidal students at the Johns Hopkins University Counseling and Student Development Center*. Unpublished doctoral dissertation, Chicago School of Professional Psychology.

Williams, M. (2001). *Suicide and attempted suicide*. London: Penguin Books.

Wingate, L. R., Joiner, T. E., Walker, R. L., Rudd, M. D., & Jobes, D. A. (2004). Empirically informed approaches to topics in suicide risk assessment. *Behavioral Science and Law, 22*, 1–15.

Wise, T. L., Jobes, D. A., Simpson, S., & Berman, A. L. (2005). *Suicidal client and clinician: Approach or avoidance*. Panel presentation at the annual conference of the American Association of Suicidology, Denver, CO.

Index

Page numbers followed by an *f* indicate figure; *t* indicate table